AF825517

# INMATE

## The Casebook Revelations of a Canadian Penitentiary Psychiatrist

# INMATE

**The Casebook Revelations of a Canadian Penitentiary Psychiatrist**

By George D. Scott, M.D. with Bill Trent

To Sharon and Al
Real Real Friends!
George Scott

**OPTIMUM PUBLISHING INTERNATIONAL INC.**
**Montreal • Toronto**

Copyright © Ottawa 1982 by Dr. George D. Scott and Bill Trent.

Population Profile Report reproduced by permission of Information Services, Correctional Services Canada.

Inmates' Rights Handbook reproduced by permission of Correctional Services Canada.

All rights reserved. No part of this book may be reproduced in any manner whatsoever without the prior written permission of the publisher.

Published by Optimum Publishing International Inc., Montréal

Legal deposit – 1st trimester 1982
Bibliothèque National du Québec

Design: Suzanne Vincent Poirier

For information contact:
Optimum Publishing International Inc.
511 Place D'Armes
Montréal, Québec
H2Y 2W7
Michael S. Baxendale, President

ISBN 0-88890-142-9

Printed and bound in Canada

*This book is respectfully dedicated to the officers of the Canadian Penitentiary Service.*

**ACKNOWLEDGMENT**

I wish to express my gratitude to the many prison colleagues and authorities who have cooperated in providing the resources used in this volume. I have been assisted particularly by Miss Susan Preen, librarian of the Correctional Staff College, Kingston; Mr. Denis Curtis, Regional Manager of Communications (Ontario); Mr. Paul Gascon, president of the Public Service Alliance, Solicitor-General Component, Ottawa; and Mr. Thomas E. Rathwell, Senior Security Officer, Ontario Region, whose thirty-four years of experience make him a valuable resource person for the crucial years from 1947 to 1981.

# FOREWORD

My late psychiatrist friend, Dr. Maurice O'Connor, stood by the fireplace, the twinkle in his eye as bright as the flames from the burning birch. "You know, fellows," he said, "there is no place in the world as interesting as a prison."

It was a Friday night in 1946 and Maurice had invited a group of us to his home in Kingston for drinks and talk about old times. Gerald Wilson was there, along with Keith McGregor, the late Earl Metcalfe and myself, all of us psychiatrists, all of us close friends. As young clinicians, we had joined the Canadian Army and served in psychiatric capacities. Now discharged, we were about to pick up the threads of our peacetime lives.

"They speak another language in prison,"Maurice pointed out. "It's really something special."

"What the hell's gotten into you?" asked Gerry, who was our senior by a few years.

What had happened was that Maurice, who had opened a private practice after discharge, had also become Kingston Penitentiary's first permanent psychiatrist – and the whole project fascinated him completely.

Psychiatry was still in its infancy in those days and we were all intrigued by it. We had what you might call the psychiatric bug and we were anxious to explore all the nooks and crannies of human behavior.

But now, imagine our much respected friend, Maurice, working inside a prison. Working inside a prisoner's mind. This, indeed, was new.

"I was surprised when somebody came to the door of my office the other day and asked if the croaker was in," Maurice said, grinning broadly. "That's what prisoners call doctors."

Maurice went on to explain that in the old days, there were no doctors attached to penitentiaries. Usually they were called from outside only when someone had died, or *croaked* as the inmates put it. Thus, they became known as *croakers*.

"They call new inmates fish," he went on. "Guards are screws."

Maurice was excited. He had immersed himself in his new milieu and was interpreting what he found psychiatrically. "Screw has a very definite emotional meaning. It's an expression of disdain for the officers."

Keith McGregor interrupted: "How do you know what's going on? Do any of the prisoners speak English?"

Maurice laughed. "I asked myself the same question when I started. But, you know, I see now that it's a very practical language they speak. Behind the walls, words often have very specific, exact and narrow meanings. There are dozens of words and expressions that mean particular things to inmates and I have to admit that there are a good many that I don't understand."

There were exciting things happening after the war. For one thing, a talented, affable Québec psychiatrist named Phil Gendreau took over the job of chief medical officer for the whole Canadian prison system. He was the first to hold a national position. Previously, medical officers had been appointed regionally. This man had big plans for revamping medical services and one of them called for the hiring of psychiatrists.

He didn't make things sound too good, either. Working inside the walls would be rough and tough. Wages would be low and guidelines would be non-existent.

That brought Gerry Wilson into the conversation again. "Does anyone know anything about prison psychiatry?" he asked. "When I went into the army, there wasn't one psychiatrist in Canada who knew the difference between an hysterical neurosis and a depressive state. In the army, nobody knew anything about psychiatry."

Keith joined the debate. "We were ignorant asses when we went into the army. We didn't know anything about anything. It took me a year before I felt I knew what I was doing."

Earl Metcalfe looked over the top of his glasses and said, "I don't think I would have the slightest bit of interest in climbing behind a wall, learning a new language and living with guys who had been crooked all their lives."

Gerry took objection to that. "I can't see a damn bit of difference between the guys behind bars and the rest of society," he said. "It's just a matter of trying to adjust to what's going on around you. If you're dealing with a bunch of people called criminals, you're dealing with nothing worse than ordinary people who got caught, or people who inadvertently found themselves involved in some kind of crime. If I worked in a prison, I think I'd get to understand people a little better."

"Maurice," I said, breaking in, "the truth is that we don't know anything about prisoners. We don't know what makes them tick. We know nothing about the psychiatric aspects of crime. We've all gotten bombed at one time or another without getting ourselves into trouble. Why do other people then get drunk and commit robberies and even kill people? Why do some people commit crimes while others do not? There are so many questions for which we have no answers."

I paused to catch my breath and noticed the room was strangely quiet. I hadn't realized that I had made a speech. The twinkle in Maurice's eye, sparked a debate among his friends. He liked doing that. He liked drawing people out, getting them to express themselves on some subject that he had introduced.

"What I meant to say is that we have no yardsticks," I put in quickly before someone else started talking. "We can't really judge human behavior. How can we know for sure that a person is mentally ill? I bet there isn't one library in Canada with information on the classification of criminals."

Maurice was a man of high principles and steeped in Catholic theology. He had read widely of the works of the thirteenth century scholar and saint, Thomas Aquinas, and had very intense feelings about good and evil.

"I just don't believe that anyone is born evil," he said.

I think Maurice knew that he was talking way above my head when he discussed the soul and how it had been created by God to form part of human existence. Man, he maintained, was composed of both soul and body.

"Thomas said the soul was interwoven with the human body," he tried to explain. "Do you understand what I mean?"

My Irish background hadn't exactly made me an expert on his favorite saint. Maurice, however, was reaching me loud and clear on the matter of prisoners. We had to stop thinking of inmates as inferior people, he said. We had to look for reasons for their actions. We had to look deeper into the question of criminality. We had to consider the crime as well as the perpetrator.

"We must not abandon our prisoners," he said. "There is so much we can do to help them and we must do it."

That was thirty-five years ago and a lot of water has passed under the proverbial bridge since. Maurice and Earl, both of whom had distinguished careers, are dead. Gerry is still in private practice in Cornwall at seventy-three years of age. Keith, who took up private practice in London, Ontario, has retired. Of the four friends who gathered in Maurice's home, I was the only one to go into penitentiary service. Officially, I am retired from the service but maintain my affiliation as psychiatric consultant at Millhaven Institution. I also have a private practice, which leaves me as busy today as I've ever been.

I often think back to that Friday night so long ago. Especially if I'm having trouble helping one of my inmate-patients cope with a particularly pressing problem. I remember how young we were then, and how green we were. Fortunately, there were people around like Maurice who not only had faith but who were able to transmit that faith to others.

I sometimes complain that we aren't moving fast enough to improve the situation of our prisons. Yet, when I look back to the early post-war years, I realize how far we've come and I think we really aren't doing all that badly.

We all owe a debt of gratitude to our early prison psychiatrists. My own debt is to Maurice O'Connor who thought that inmates should be regarded as people – and to Thomas Aquinas who taught Maurice about good and evil.

A final note: Although the facts and events described in this book are based on actual criminal histories, most of the individuals who appear in them are identified by fictitious first names. This has been done so as not to violate the anonymity many of these subjects require to assure their successful rehabilitation. Actual names have only been used in highly publicized cases in which that anonymity no longer exists. Care has also been taken to avoid pinpointing specific locations where this may do harm to individuals.

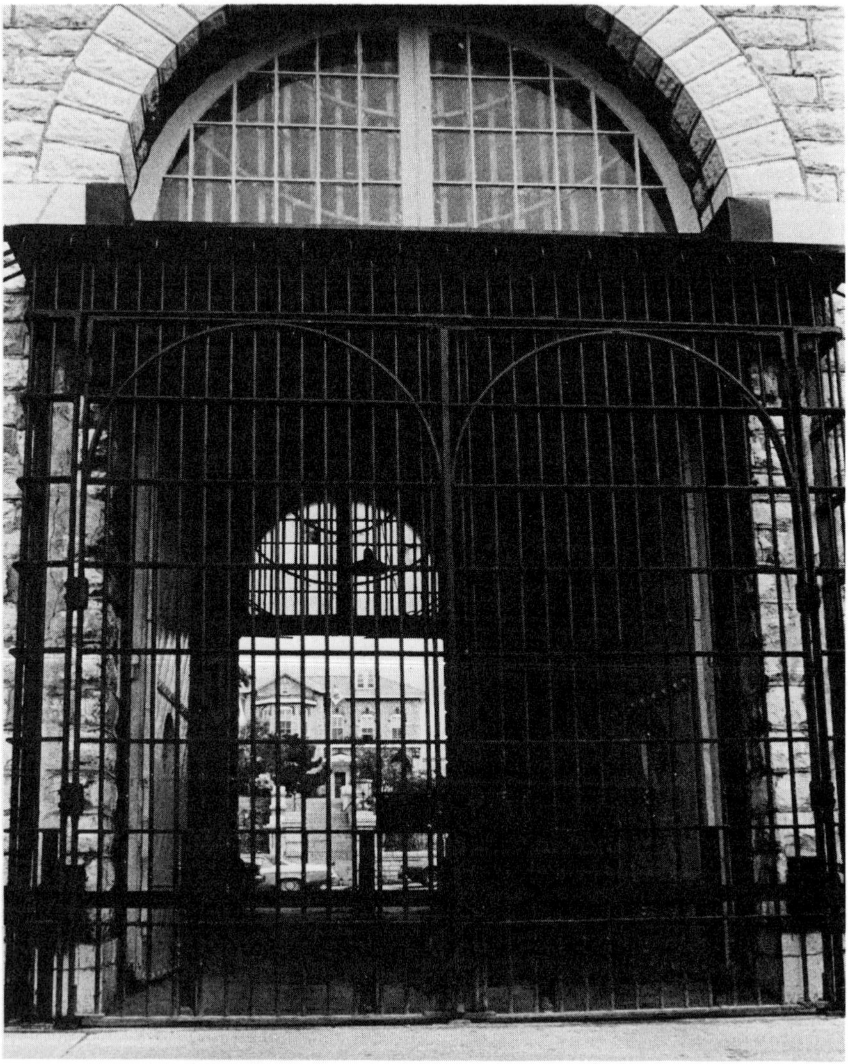

*The North Gate at Kingston Penitentiary.*
*This gate is the only passageway between freedom and captivity.*

*(Barry Wright)*

ERRATA

Chapter 4 should read The Prison Subculture
Chapter 5 should read Psychiatric Syndromes in Prison
Chapter 6 should read Millhaven: The Super-Maximum Prison
Chapter 7 should read Hostage-taking: A Sucker's Game
Chapter 8 should read The Criminal Personality
The Publishers regret the error.

## CONTENTS:


| | | |
|---|---|---|
| | Foreword | IX |
| **Chapter 1** | Case History of a Sexual Psychopath | 1 |
| **Chapter 2** | Bloody Sunday | 9 |
| **Chapter 3** | The Riot: Why? | 17 |
| **Chapter 4** | Millhaven: The Super-Maximum Prison | 22 |
| **Chapter 5** | Hostage-taking: A Sucker's Game | 30 |
| **Chapter 6** | The Criminal Personality | 35 |
| **Chapter 7** | The Prison Subculture | 39 |
| **Chapter 8** | Psychiatric Syndromes in Prison | 47 |
| **Chapter 9** | Murderers I Have Known | 65 |
| **Chapter 10** | Murder in the Early, Middle and Later Years | 68 |
| **Chapter 11** | Insanity Pleas | 87 |
| **Chapter 12** | Psychiatry in Court | 99 |
| **Chapter 13** | Suicides, Slashings and Other Stories | 105 |
| **Chapter 14** | Special Cases | 117 |
| **Chapter 15** | Brew Masters | 125 |
| **Chapter 16** | Drugs: Highs and Lows Behind the Walls | 130 |
| **Chapter 17** | The Prison For Women | 137 |
| **Chapter 18** | Michael and Sean Were Sweethearts | 157 |
| **Chapter 19** | An Experiment in Sensory Deprivation | 166 |
| **Chapter 20** | Crime Denial and Confession | 174 |
| **Chapter 21** | Steven Truscott: A Personal Investigation | 181 |
| **Chapter 22** | Guards: Front-Line Story | 188 |
| **Chapter 23** | Reward City: A New Penal Environment | 195 |
| **Appendix I** | Population Profile Report | 203 |
| **Appendix II** | Inmates' Rights Handbook | 207 |

# CHAPTER 1

## Case History of a Sexual Psychopath

In the Central Registry of the penitentiaries division of the federal department of the Solicitor-General in Ottawa lies a file bulging with notes, observations, parole applications, letters, psychological assessments and psychiatric reports on one of the most sex-tormented individuals I have seen in my penitentiary practice. He was a strange man with a bizarre view of life whom I shall call John.

The word "DEAD" has been stamped on his file – but his memory lives on among all of us who knew him in penitentiary. He is a classic example of the proverbial lost cause; yet everyone on the penal team hoped he could be saved.

They hoped it to the bitter, violent end.

John lived in a world of fantasy and his fantasies were peopled by girls. Young girls, usually. Very young. And sometimes he wrote stories about them.

"A Day in the Country" was one of those stories.

"She had nice long blonde hair, deep blue eyes, lips like cherries and her skin was like cream," he wrote. "She wore a white blouse, a bright red skirt that barely came to her knees and white shorts and running shoes."

He became almost poetic in his perversion as he described how his imaginary little girl walked and how her movements aroused him sexually.

"A Day in the Country" told a lot about John.

"It was on a very hot summer Sunday afternoon in July when I thought I would take a walk into the woods. The path I walked along was lonely and baren, leading me further into the woods."

"I was about five hundred yards in when I heard somebody coming from up ahead. As the person approached me from the distance, I stopped...wondering what anyone was doing out here all alone. As I approached, I noticed that it was a little girl of not more than 7 or 8 years old and she was dragging a tricycle along. I said what's wrong with your bike. Hi.. she said, I got a damn twisted wheel. Hey, that's not nice language for a nice cute little girl to use. Well, I ain't nice and if you had to push this damn bike you would swear too. Here, let me fix it for you. O.K. thank you and I will give you a nice big kiss afterwards or do anything you want to do. I know of a nice place we can go to fix it down along the creek a ways and nobody can see us or bother us."

He writes about taking the girl to a cool, shady place where there is a lawn and a swimming hole and suggests that she go swimming while he fixes her bike. She has no swimsuit, so she goes into the water in her skirt.

"When she took her blouse off, I nearly blew my stones. What a sweet body she had and her little nipples so pink. What's your name? Mine is John. 'Betty.' 'How old are you Betty?' I'm 7 almost 8. 'How old are you?' 'Oh, just about 19.' Betty went swimming and I worked on the wheel and when I finished I called Betty out and said, 'All done.' Now where is that big kiss?' She didn't say anything but put her wet arms around my neck and put her lips on mine. So I put my arms around her bare body and pulled her to me and kissed her hard and long..."

He goes into a minute description of his sexual encounter with the little girl, making it amply clear that she is enjoying the experience as much as he. The thought of a nineteen-year-old having sexual relations with a child of seven is, of course, revolting. John doesn't see it that way. His day in the country is, quite simply, idyllic.

John's story is an ugly story.

It's also frightening.

One has to dig deep into John's background, however, to see what made him tick and to understand the strange drama that would be unfolding later in Kingston Penitentiary.

John was a very dangerous man. He was a sexual psychopath.

John was born in 1944, the third of eight children. His father was a tradesman and his parents remembered him as a sickly baby, different from other children. He would not react to scolding as did his brothers and sister and frequently had temper tantrums, "running all over people's property." He was often afraid to ask for things and frequently appeared guilty and fearful. Until he was sixteen, his parents controlled him with a "good licking." When he got older, they were unable to handle him. At home and at school, he tended to be a lone wolf. He left school during Grade 8 after a sexual incident with a female pupil.

John first ran afoul of the law in August 1960, when he took a nine-year-old girl into a church and tried to remove her jeans. (He was sixteen.) This, he did several times, until the girl's older sister arrived and told him to leave her alone. Taken into custody, he was sent to the Ontario Hospital for observation, then put on probation.

In October 1960, he needed money and broke into a home. Two months later, he entered a girls' washroom in the public school he attended and "annoyed" a Grade 7 female student. He was convicted of break-and-entry on the first offence and of breach of probation in the case of the girl and sent to the Ontario Reformatory at Guelph.

He was discharged from Guelph on October 6, 1962. The very next day he succumbed to his desires to fondle minors. A few days later, he was in court, charged with indecent assault on four girls, aged three, four, five and six. Hamilton magistrate W. R. Morrison, gave him two years on these charges. He also found him guilty of being a dangerous sexual offender and sentenced him to an indefinite term of preventive detention.

John entered Kingston Penitentiary with two strikes against him. First, he was being incarcerated for a period which could be as long as his life, depending on the progress he made. Second, he was going into an openly hostile environment, prison inmates having a notorious dislike of anyone involved in sexual offences with children.

S. M. Farrell, K.P.'s supervisor of classification at the time, entered him into his report as a youth who looked younger than his eighteen years, with a facial rash that left him with a generalized condition of pimples.

John was candid and frank in all discussions concerning his sex problems and home life. He said his first remembered sex incident was with his younger sister who was eight years old at the time. He fondled her in much the same way as he would fondle other girls later. When she refused to comply, he stopped. He was shy and insecure with girls his own age and thus had never acquired any girl friends. He never engaged in intercourse. He admitted wearing female undergarments and said he became very excited when he did. Sometimes, too, he watched his sister and mother undress. On one occasion, he recalled, he bore a hole in the floor of his mother's room, so that he could look up at her from the basement.

He was a pathetic youth when I first met him in consultation. Our interviews were labored and difficult. He was anything but alert intellectually and I had to address him in a slow and obvious way. He told me about marital discord in his family. His parents had never had a settled existence and he reflected that instability. He was quite attached to his mother but less so to his father, who had warned him in no uncertain terms after his first conviction that he didn't want him around the house.

John ran into trouble almost as soon as he walked into the pen. One of the more aggressive inmates walked over to him and said, "Hey, creep, you wanna play with somebody's crotch?" John backed away. "You ain't gonna find no three-year-old girl in this joint."

It was obvious from the outset that the inmates were going to exact their own brand of punishment on John. "Fucking pervert," one strong-arm inmate was heard to say, lifting his middle finger into the air as an obscene gesture. "We're gonna fuck you good." There were many encounters like this and sometimes two or three inmates would fall in around him and smash their fists into his stomach until he reeled under the pain. Once, somebody brought his knee up into his groin. John was sick to his stomach for two days after that.

For his own safety, John was put in segregation soon after his arrival. He was given a cell in an area of the prison reserved for sexual offenders, who are constantly harrassed by other inmates, and for other outcasts of the inmate population, who are often equally bothered – stool pigeons.

"He is presently in segregation where he has been placed for his own protection," I wrote in a memorandum to the warden and other officials in 1963. "He presents the picture of an unaspiring adolescent who is the object of the blows of his more aggressive inmates who seem to punish him for his assaults on young girls."

We know that symptoms of aberrant behavior often show up early in life. The problem is that so often we don't do anything about them, though I have to admit, of course, that it's usually easier to do what's right when one is an outsider, unaffected by the emotions of a situation.

It was known at home that John spent his leisure time reading sexually stimulating literature and that he carried clippings from girlie magazines in his pockets. It was known that he masturbated frequently, an act which his mother described as "fooling around with himself." It was known that he kept items of women's wear under the mattress of his bed. On one occasion, when he was arrested, he was wearing women's underpants.

John's mother (and indeed his father) knew there was something wrong. The transvestite problem alone needed attention. But his parents failed to communicate with the authorities. Instead, John was urged by his mother to practice faith as an approach to solving his problem. He took the advice and joined a Christian Scientist group. It was an association that failed to provide him with a solution.

John was put through a barrage of tests in prison. The Raven's Progressive Matrices Test rated his intellectual capacity as "definitely below average." His Rorschach test (for personality analysis) revealed that his personality development had been "highly disturbed" in his early years.

Fixated, immature sexual attitudes were noted throughout testing. He showed a marked inability to control his emotional reactions. Affection-seeking existed to a disproportionate degree, and although he consciously defended himself from his own impulses by repression, the mechanism seemed to have totally failed to prevent aberrant behavior.

In 1964, he was showing some apparent improvement. At one point, he told a parole officer that if he believed he would be unable to conduct himself in a proper way outside prison, he might as well stay behind bars for the rest of his life. This was interpreted as meaning he was trying to contend with his problem in some way.

He was coping with another problem, too. A Parole Service report made known: "He states that he has never indulged in homosexual activities in the institution. He states that never as long as he is here will he ever do it. He is under pressure from more aggressive inmates to be a sex partner but it is his claim that he has never given in. His sexual outlet is masturbation."

The report added this bright note: "This man's outlook is in the process of changing."

Some time later, John made an application for parole. In his own simple way, he opened his remarks with an apology. "Dear sirs," he wrote, "sorry to bother you but I'd like if possible to win back my freedom." He said he had gotten into trouble because he hung around with the wrong friends. He now felt he could start life over again as a normal man. "All I am asking," he said, "is one last chance to prove to you that I've been cured." His application was deferred.

It was clear to me that John's weak mental ability prevented him from having any insight into his own deviant thinking. Psychotherapy, I was forced to conclude, was pointless and incarceration was the only safe way in which to protect society from his sexual aberrations.

John's life didn't improve with the passing of time. He was let out of segregation and given work in the carpentry shop but he was shunned by the other inmates. Then his cell was searched and officers found a book with pictures of young children pasted in it. They also found pictures of nude women and a book containing obscene stories he had written. Later, he was given minor offence reports for disobeying orders.

During one of my interviews, John complained that he had lost his recreational privileges and wanted them back. I reminded him that he had been writing dirty stories and drawing filthy pictures in his cell.

"Well, Doc," he replied in a kind of drawl, "it's like smoking. It gets to be a habit." Once again, he was reinforcing my belief that there was no hope from a psychiatric point of view of ever changing him.

In 1966, he re-applied for parole. He wrote: "I have reason to think that I won't repeat my crime because I understand more fully ... the consequences of this crime and fully realize that if I am given a parole and do commit this particular crime that I would never probably get another chance cause this will be my third try." The request was turned down.

In a later report, Parole Service representative L. W. Hunt said: "This is a most pathetic case. (The subject) is a very nervous person at this time. While waiting for an answer to a question, he will click his teeth or suck in his breath with a loud noise."

John told Hunt he would not reject sex after release from prison because this would not be normal. However, he said he would go with girls of his own age. He was quoted in Hunt's report as saying: "When I masturbate now, I think of women instead of young girls. I've been doing this for the past year."

Hunt was moved by the interview. "He certainly gives the impression of being a very lonely and sensitive lad," he wrote. "He impresses me as a very simple and suggestive person who very badly wants and needs someone to try and understand or help him." He thought he would be better off in a mental institution where he could receive attention from "people who understand this type of person."

In 1967, John was concerned with the significance of his dreams, which were mostly sexual in nature. Up until then, a girl under the age of ten had filled his dreams. He remembered "living it up with a little girl in an apartment." Now, however, males were dominating the sexual activities in his dreams and he was afraid he had become a homosexual. He wrote letters to other inmates in which he suggested encounters for mutual sexual gratification, describing in detail the methods he would employ and which he would expect them to use. He claimed that he had never had the opportunity to join in a homosexual act in the pentitentiary but that he would if he had the chance.

John was no closer to parole in 1967 than he had been in 1962. Peter R. Cotton, classification officer, wrote in a report: "It is rather sad that the writer must make the same recommendation year after year but the subject is simply not ready for parole."

In 1970, John's sex life was an active one. He admitted to considerable homosexual activity, playing both active and passive roles. He also admitted that he masturbated frequently, often three times a day, with sexual fantasies involving both males and females with an age spread of between ten and thirty-five years. He had given up writing stories like "A Day in the Country" but still collected pictures of little girls.

His sexual urges were insatiable.

In an appraisal report in July, 1970, Parole Service Officer, D. M. Stienburg said John remained the "same pitifully inadequate" man of earlier reports. He added, "He functions like a child and, I feel, is totally incapable of functioning in an acceptable manner in free society."

On September 15, John appeared before a National Parole Board panel at the penitentiary. At this point, he had served eight years of his preventive detention sentence. He told the panel that he had made some effort to gain a better understanding of himself and had been reading books to increase his knowledge and self-confidence. The most recent book he had read was "The Power of Positive Thinking" by Norman Vincent Peale and he believed this had helped him.

He said he now felt he would be able to handle himself adequately in the community. The panel didn't think he could. Its members agreed that he showed some improvement but felt he still was not ready for release. They deferred parole to October 30, 1971.

But that date was going to be too late for John.

* * *

On April 14, 1971, Kingston Penitentiary's more than eight hundred inmates launched one of the most violent riots in Canadian penal history. In a 90-hour rampage, they virtually demolished their entire living quarters in the main cell block, causing more than $1.5 million damage. For six officers taken hostage, it was the most frightening experience of their lives. The most bizarre event of the whole rumble, however, occurred on the last day of the riot, Sunday April 18.

They called it Bloody Sunday. It was the day the rioters went after the undesirables in the prison population: child molesters, rapists, perverts, stoolies – mostly emotional offenders. It was, one inmate said, a kind of "day of atonement" for the outcasts.

Inmates clammed up after the incident – as they always do. It's part of the inmate code: you don't turn informer, no matter what. But the story came out, in bits and pieces.

They came storming into the segregation area, a dozen of them, perhaps more, armed with steel bars. They smashed the locking mechanism and opened the doors of the cells. There were frightened screams from the occupants, and fiendish catcalls from the attackers.

John was cowering in the corner of his cell when they came, the safety and security of segregation now nothing more than a myth.

"Hey, diddler," one of the inmates called out, beckoning him with a fast-twitching index finger.

"Outside, creep," another inmate ordered.

John got up and stepped out of the cell. He was surrounded by a number jeering inmates.

"You man or woman, pervert?" somebody asked.

"You the fucker or the fuckee?" another laughed.

John's drawl was slower than usual. "Where we goin'?" he asked.

"We're goin' to a party," one of the men replied. "We got a real nice party for you. Only maybe you won't think so. You see..." The inmate winked at one of his cohorts and started to laugh. "You see, there ain't gonna be no little girls there."

## CHAPTER 2

# Bloody Sunday

Kingston Penitentiary (K.P.) sits squarely on sixteen and a half acres of the best prime land on Lake Ontario, described in the cadastral lists as Lot No. 20 in the first concession of the township of Kingston. It is surrounded by four great limestone walls, twenty-five feet in height, surmounted by four observation towers, one at each corner, manned by armed guards around the clock to ensure perimeter security. It was conceived in 1833 as an impregnable fortress for the captive society, built to withstand the winds of the lake – and of time.

The walls enclose a number of buildings, the largest of which is the main cell block, where the inmate population is housed. One of the original buildings, it was constructed in basic cruciform design, the four bars of which comprise cell blocks running north, south, east and west from a large central area known as the "dome." The building actually is crowned by a dome, built cathedral-style. It once had windows (now boarded over) to provide light in the days before electricity.

The four cell blocks radiating from the dome were designed to quarter the population in individual cells. Each block is four levels high and there are four stairways leading to them. At each level, a narrow passageway runs around the perimeter of the dome, bound by a waist-high handrail but otherwise open to the dome area. Each floor of the blocks is known as a "range."

In the middle of the nineteenth century, the old stone fortress echoed with the anguished cries of its inhabitants, many of whom were children. Women and children were flogged with merciless abandon in those days (Peter Charbonneau, for instance, was only ten when he was lashed fifty-seven times for childish acts of disobedience) and their cries were heard across the walls and in the streets of the town.

There were anguished cries and frightened screams across the walls in April of 1971 too, but these were the sounds of insurrection.

Security had always been tight at K.P. It was tight this mild Wednesday evening. It was a matter of pride to officials and staff that no one had broken out in the last decade. Security was a way of life. Cell to mess hall, mess hall to cell. Cell to shop, shop to cell. Cell to recreation area, recreation area to cell. Every inmate move was regimented and watched over by men with guns.

And still it happened.

Don Flynn is a big, heavy-set man with one of those knuckle-cracking handshakes, a strong commanding voice and the unmistakeable air of a former military man. He's still erect and clipped in his mannerisms but has grown somewhat paunchy in the years since he left the armed services. But he still looks as though he might have been a sergeant-major at one time. In fact, he was a private in the Hastings and Prince Edward Infantry in the Second World War and fought in Italy. He spins a good war yarn over vodka and water at the Legion. He tells even better stories about the old pen and the night they beat the shit out of the sex offenders.

Don was senior correctional officer and a penal service veteran of twenty-two years at K.P. when the riot broke out. Later, he was posted to Millhaven Institution, a prison built in the early seventies to replace K.P. as Ontario's major maximum security centre. After surviving ninety terrifying hours as one of six hostages in the riot, and then going through some sixty disturbances at Millhaven, he decided he'd had enough and retired.

Don isn't one of those people who enjoys pulling out at age fifty-five. He left the prison service because he'd had it up to here. I don't see him as much now as I used to but he comes in every so often, sometimes to chew the fat, other times to renew his prescription for Librium. He doesn't take the pills regularly. Only when he feels the need of them. They quieten his stomach, he says, and ease his nerves.

Don has had a pretty rough time of it over the last few years. He used to be steady as a rock. He could put his hand out palm down after five or six vodkas and you wouldn't see so much as a finger move. Now, he gets uptight easily. His face becomes taut as he talks about the pen. He clenches and unclenches his fists.

Don faced what he thought was certain death during the riot and this is not the kind of thing a man forgets easily. He began having dreams, bad dreams. In his dreams he is up on the fourth range, up near the top of the dome, and the inmates are grabbing him and pulling him over to the railing on the walkway. Then suddenly, he feels himself going over the railing. He's about to plunge down the seventy feet to the concrete floor below when he wakes up.

Don still has dreams, though they are not as bad as they once were, and he doesn't mind talking about them. The last one he told me about concerned a real knockdown fight:

"I'm fighting these eight guys. I don't know who. Rioters, I guess they are. There's a terrible struggle. I'm up against a wall, then down on the ground. I let go with a left hook and all of a sudden all hell breaks loose and Eileen is screaming, 'Wake up, Don, for God's sake wake up.' I sit up and I'm in a dead sweat. I've been punching the bedclothes all to hell, as I do many nights. Only this time I've landed this punch right on Eileen's shoulder and I look at her and Jesus, I don't know if she's going to cry or what."

Don, who had been working the four p.m. to midnight shift, was one of the first to become involved in the riot. In his statement to officials later, he said he had gone to the centre of the dome to supervise the movement of inmates from the recreation area to their cells. Suddenly, several inmates rushed the area, attacking him and Keeper Edward Barrett, officer in charge of the evening shift.

"They grabbed us and threw me on the floor," he said. "I struggled and gave up when I was overpowered by the number of inmates." Don and Barrett were hustled into a corridor where they were joined by four other officers who had been taken hostage. Later, an inmate arrived and demanded the hostages' watches and money. Don gave him his Timex watch and ten dollars. After this, the hostages were moved from one location to another. At one point, they were ordered to remove their clothing and don inmate garb. This way, the rioters figured, if there was any shooting, the outside guards wouldn't know whom they were shooting.

Through most of the riot, Flynn and his co-workers were protected by a group of inmates who had been given this as an assignment. They did their job well. One of them provided the group with contraband soup, which he had stolen earlier and stashed away. Another brought cigarettes and razors.

The first hours of the disturbance had been reasonably calm but by the following day, things were getting tense. The rioters shouted catcalls and banged on the steel guard rails on the walkways with steel bars. At one point, several hundred inmates banged incessantly on the rails for several minutes. The pounding created fierce echoes that virtually deafened those near the top of the dome.

The rioting was confined to the main cell block, but in the psychiatric unit, located in a building just across a walkway, my one hundred and ten patients were tense. They knew what was going on and some of them were hiding behind their beds for safety. Had the disturbance spilled over into the unit, I'm sure they would have run amok. I gave them capsules of chloral hydrate, so they could sleep.

On the second day in the main building, the rioters were running wild. They were equipped with steel bars, knives and home-made spears. Their victims now were the institution's young inmates who, frightened for their lives, hid in the ducts. The older rioters found them and raped them, there on the spot, or out in the dome area.

"The queers really had a ball," Don Flynn made known later. "They reamed this one guy so hard he couldn't walk. He was a kid. Maybe seventeen or eighteen. This other kid, though...he was raped so many times, his rectum just flopped out."

As riots go, the insurrection of April, 1971 was one of the most serious – if not the most serious – in the then 135-year history of K.P. By the time it was over, one man would be dead, a second dying, thirteen would be wounded and whole areas of the prison destroyed. Even the walls between cells would be smashed. Much of the havoc the inmates wreaked is still in evidence today, whole sections of the big cell block having been left in ruins.

It was a major riot, no doubt about it. It was also one of the most bizarre. Nobody is really quite sure why it happened and nobody knows why, at its height, rampaging inmates went after sexual offenders. Except that hard core inmates – aggressive, physical individuals such as bank robbers – hate so-called emotional offenders. The aggressives will understand a man who kills his wife. After all, he may have had good reason. But a *diddler*, a man who enjoys sexual play with a child? He is perverted and deserves anything he gets.

In the early hours of Sunday morning, April 18, the strange circus got started. It would leave a number of experienced officers in a state of shock. It was something that every officer in the penitentiary would remember for the rest of his life.

Bloody Sunday. It was the day we thought the *straights* had gone after the *weirdos*. Don Flynn corrected this. Some of the straights, he said, weren't all that straight. Whatever their inclinations, a roving group of them went looking for victims. They found fifteen of them in segregation cells, most crouching in abject fear on the floor beside their bunks. They were trapped.

The rioters dragged their victims, some of them screaming, from the cells. They pulled and pushed them along the corridor to the centre of the dome area. Rioters on other tiers yelled obscenities down on the victims. There had been a good catch in segregation that day – rapists, child molesters and a variety of other perverts. Not all, however, were sexual offenders. Some of those in segregation were there because they had had trouble with other inmates. One, for instance, had reportedly run afoul of the strong-arm boys over an unpaid gambling debt.

They set up chairs, fifteen of them, in a circle and tied their victims to them. Fifteen chairs for fifteen undesirables. It could have been a re-enactment of an ancient Druid ritual, or more appropriately perhaps, a scene from a horror movie. Then they draped sheets over them, white sheets they had ripped off the beds in their victims' cells, covering them from head to foot.

And the show began.

It was a kangaroo court, the outcasts of the penitentiary culture being judged and punished by their peers. A bank robber named Karl was the judge and he dispensed "justice." There was a jury, too, but its members were also the executioners. They moved around the circle of chairs in a ghoulish kind of ritual, letting out a stream of catcalls and invectives that reverberated around the old limestone walls and echoed in a spiral that reached the very top of the dome.

Don Flynn got a running account of events from a twenty-eight-year-old robber named Scott, a member of the inmate team set up to protect the hostages. It was he who had provided the contraband soup. Scott kept going down to the "court" area to see what was going on.

Scott was tense when he got back from one of his visits below. "Them crazy bastards down there," he said, "they've got those guys tied up and they're trying them." He shook his head, as though he was having trouble believing his own words.

Don Flynn couldn't see the floor of the dome from where he was but he could hear the voice of the man with the megaphone. The man was yelling into the instrument and much of what he said was distorted. Don could hear him distinctly, however, when he pronounced the verdicts. "He's guilty," were words that were repeated several times. Guilty of what? Guilty of being *creeps*.

The men signalled their approval of the "trials" by banging on the guard rails and shouting. But they became strangely quiet when one of the accused spoke up in his defence. "Goddamn bastards," he said. "What did I ever do to you?" There was a moment of silence and then his voice broke into a roar. "Goddamn bastards, Goddamn bastards." There was another moment of quiet and then he said, "Why me? You committed crimes as bad as mine. Bastards... "

Don recognized the voice. It was that of an inmate with whom he had had considerable contact over the years. It was John. John, the quiet, shy, retiring child molester. He had come in like a lamb and now he was roaring like a lion. "He yelled so loud they must have heard him on the streets downtown," Don would tell fellow officers later.

John's words were soon smothered in catcalls from the ranges. The inmates had gathered by the score around the walkways, peering down on the show below. It was standing room only in the gallery, but the view was unobstructed.

The jurymen carried steel bars – the very steel bars that had kept the prisoners in their cell blocks. The really strong men among them had literally torn the bars from their door frames in an incredible display of enraged strength. (Prison officials, inspecting the damage after the riot, were at a loss to explain how the inmates had managed to bend and twist the bars to the point where they could wrest them from their frames. Yet, wrest them they had.)

The jurymen-cum-executioners, their faces contorted, their eyes wild, their lips parted in ugly grimaces, according to inmate accounts, then did their dirty work. They raised their steel bars and brought them down on their victims, squirming and screaming under the sheets, and as they moved about the circle, they continued their attacks. They struck with angry force. They struck their heads and their shoulders. They struck their backs and their chests. They beat them on the arms and on the legs. Nobody knows exactly how many blows were delivered.

While the inmates continued to riot inside, soldiers from the Canadian Forces base at nearby Barriefield held positions on the grounds of the institution, waiting for a command to move in. They had been called by a seasoned warden, Art Jarvis, some time earlier. For the hostages, the presence of the army was a kind of mixed blessing. On the one hand, it was good to know that help was that close. On the other hand, it had made the inmates jittery as they felt an armed assault was imminent.

Then, in the midst of the melee, three men from the "hostage protector" group surrounded Don. "You, hit it, let's go," one of them said, jerking the thumb of his right hand back to indicate the range corridor. Don didn't know why they had selected him in particular from among the six hostages, but he didn't argue. He figured he had been marked for execution.

"I said goodbye to my friends and we all shook hands," Don would relate after. "It was very solemn. They wished me good luck but I knew what they were thinking. They were thinking this was it, too. And maybe they'd be next. It's a strange feeling, thinking you're going to die.

Don took a few steps along the corridor with his escort and another inmate from the protector group intercepted. "Where the hell you takin' this guy?" he asked. "We're taking the son of a bitch down below," the escort replied. "You're not takin' him nowhere," the first man snapped back. "One of these guys gets hurt and we're wiped out. The army'll walk in and there won't be one of us alive."

Don was pretty shook up after that. Supposing, he began to think, supposing some of the inmates decided to slip him over the railing. Rumors had already circulated that some of the militants were going to rush the hostages. It was a sheer drop of seventy feet to the floor of the dome and there wouldn't be much left of him when he hit the ground. Don remembered the men who had jumped to their deaths there over the years and he shuddered.

That's when Don made the bargain with his friendly protector, Scott. Don remembers the conversation well:

"If they try to put me over the railing, you make sure you get me before I go," Don quotes himself as saying. "I mean, kill me. Knife, anything. Just be sure I'm dead before I go over."

Scott listened quietly, his eyes riveted on Don's face as he spoke. "I sure as hell will, boss," Scott said earnestly, his face displaying concern for his captive. "You always used me right."

Scott and Don never had to put the bargain to the test. That Sunday afternoon, the disturbance came to an end, a plan for the release of the hostages and return of the inmates to normal custody having been worked out by members of an inmate committee and a citizens' committee composed of four prominent lawyers and a media personality. The latter body, under the chairmanship of noted legal authority Arthur Martin, Q.C., included lawyers William R. Donkin, J. Desmond Morton, Q.C., and Aubrey E. Golden, and columnist-author Ron Haggart.

Because K.P. had been so heavily damaged, a great many inmates found themselves without cell accommodations. These men were transferred to other area institutions, notably the new maximum security penitentiary at Millhaven, fifteen miles away to the west.

The riot resulted in court appearances for a number of inmates, extra time added to sentences and close confinement for twelve men believed to be the ringleaders. They were dispatched to Millhaven's super maximum Special Handling Unit where they became known as "The Dirty Dozen." The riot also resulted in the naming of a commission of inquiry under the chairmanship of Vancouver lawyer J.W. Swackhamer, Q.C., which considered a voluminous "fundamental instability" in the prison system.

Don Flynn's position as senior correctional officer gave him access to many sources of information but details of that strange "trial" in the dome were scant. The inmates had suddenly all come down with laryngitis. Don recalls trying to get information from an inmate, a sixty-five-year-old *diddler* from way back, immediately after the riot was over. "Rebellious old devil," Don said. "He had cuts and bruises all over his head. He was a mess. But he'd never whine about anything. When I tried to talk to him, he just laughed and said, 'First one to the showers'."

Don's inquiries, however, did produce some information.

As the victims of the "court" collapsed under their attackers' blows, their bodies were dragged into a corridor. At the conclusion of the "trial," the fifteen men lay limp, one on top of the other, in a huge human pile.

Someone in the mound then whispered a warning to the man on top of him. The warning was repeated a number of times to other victims. It was a simple admonition: play dead; don't move a muscle. And no one did. They lay absolutely still for nearly a whole day, the inmates on the bottom of the pile close to suffocation under the pressure of bodies.

Only once during that day did the executioners come over to where the bodies lay. It was to find John. He was near the top of the heap, only semi-conscious.

"We'd better finish the little fucker off," someone said.

And someone did.

**CHAPTER 3**

# The Riot: Why?

Inmate stabbings are commonplace in our penitentiaries, so commonplace that even a news-hungry media considers four killings in as many months at Millhaven routine copy. Suicides happen often enough to be ignored by journalists unless there are unusually interesting extenuating circumstances. Now, hostage-taking has become a major feature of many disturbances, an extremely dangerous development since hostages are not necessarily people performing custodial duties.

Riots, protests, sit-downs, slow-downs – they're happening with alarming frequency in our penal institutions. In British Columbia, New Brunswick, Québec, Ontario. Virtually everywhere.

What the hell's going on in our penitentiaries?

I am not as critical of our correctional structure as some. I don't despair every time a problem arises. In general terms, in fact, I believe our prison system works rather efficiently. The term "maximum security," however, has become synonymous with violence in the minds of many people, and not without reason. Maximum security institutions do tend to be the centre of violence. When a major disturbance occurs, it is almost certain to be in one of the top security prisons, not in minimum or medium security centres.

Obviously, there has to be something wrong somewhere.

The old hard-line prison philosophy is still alive among many people. You still hear custodial officers say things like "lock the bastards up and throw away the keys."

Many, like Don Flynn, would like to see the return of corporal and capital punishment. "When you gave a guy the strap, the other troublemakers thought twice about causing a disturbance," he says. "And knowing you could be hanged for murder made you cautious about running a *shiv* (a knife) into a guard."

But that's old time penal religion.

They no longer call Kingston Penitentiary the College of Criminal Knowledge. It once was the institution to which boys in reformatories graduated when they came of age. Indeed, many of them aspired to it. But the day of great stone fortresses for great masses of offenders is past. In 1975, K.P., antiquated, inadequate and left in virtual ruins by the big riot of '71, became two separate centres: the Regional Reception Centre, where new inmates are classified and sent on to other institutions, and the Regional Psychiatric Centre.

Kingston Penitentiary, as many people still refer to it, hasn't lost its glamor. It's still "The Big House" and it still accommodates some five hundred men, counting inmates being processed, those who are there in protective custody, and psychiatric patients.

But the reformatory kids who graduate to adult institutions today don't contemplate places like K.P. They want places with amenities, man.

Criminology has moved into a new era. Punishment in a modern prison is really indirect. Floggings have been banned and "hard labor" is an archaic term meaning, for all practical purposes, nothing. Punishment, in effect, is the act of being in prison, of being deprived of one's freedom. Treatment and rehabilitation have come of age. You need only attend a magistrate's court, or a meeting of a legal group associated with sentencing, to recognize that today the sentence is really the initiation – hopefully anyway – of a treatment process.

A good many changes have taken place in our penal system. You seldom hear inmates complaining about the food anymore. Why would they? They eat better than many people on the outside. You don't hear many complaints about lice-ridden bedding and rat-infested cells anymore either because accommodations have been improved enormously in recent years. Inmates once were forbidden to talk to one another, except with permission. There is no longer such a rule. Today, they work together in art classes, participate in group therapy, take part in group discussions. Inmates once were expected to obey every rule blindly, without questions. Today, inmate committees take up all kinds of grievances with the administration, much as unions do in the outside world.

Collins Bay, on the outskirts of Kingston, has numerous amenities for inmates, among them color television in some cells. The inmates react positively. They call it "Disneyland." "You know why they call it that, don't you?" an old-time correctional man says. "Because it's a fun place. They got everything there but women."

You can't call Millhaven a fun place. The inmates will tell you it's a tough nut of a joint. But if you can get into the farm annex, you've got it made. They've even got a nine-hole golf course out there.

So, what are they beefing about, the hardliners want to know?

In Kingston Penitentiary in 1971, they were beefing about a lot of things, among them boredom, sheer unadulterated boredom, the kind of absolute boredom that sends some inmates screaming up the walls. There is boredom in our institutions today and it can be devastating. There are times when just the very fact that a man is in prison, that he sits in a cell with bars, that he can't go out on the street and see people, is enough to send him into a depression.

I listen to a lot of people who are very upset about the simple fact of their confinement. This break-and-entry patient was extremely agitated on one recent visit to my office.

"In about five seconds, Doc, I'm going right through that window," he said pointing over this shoulder to a solid wall.

"Bobby," I said. "I want to tell you something. There's no window back there. Just wall."

Bobby thought for a moment and then he said, "I'm going through anyway."

* * *

The Swackhamer inquiry into the riot at K.P. was an exhaustive one and its recommmendations far-reaching. If it's possible to learn something from a riot, I think this may be a case in point.

The inquiry could find no single identifiable cause of the disturbance but concluded that it had been the result of a system that had failed because of its inability to establish and maintain a strong rehabilitative program. Among possible supporting causes, it referred to such things as the aged physical facilities of K.P., overcrowding, the shortage of professional staff, an activity program that had been substantially curtailed, confinement of people who did not require maximum security, too much time spent in cells, lack of adequate channels to deal with complaints and lack of adequate staff to deal with inmate requests.

The objectives of a penitentiary are to hold the individual in custody for the period of his sentence, and to prepare him to return to the community to live as a law-abiding and contributing citizen. Each is of equal importance. The inability to attain either is a sign of failure on the part of the institution. How to keep both objectives in balance is the prison dilemma. It's obvious that failure to achieve an adequate custodial system will pose danger for the community and certainly brings the administration of justice into disrepute. Failure to create and maintain a program sufficient to prepare an individual for his return to the community poses equal danger in the long run however, increasing recidivism, with substantial damage to the community. The inquiry was particularly concerned with what it termed the "depressing and dehumanizing" effects of confinement. From a psychiatrist's point of view, this was getting down to fundamentals.

Psychiatrists come under a lot of fire from time to time. We're told we're bleeding hearts because we try to help inmates in the rehabilitative process. We're told we would be making better use of our time if we concerned ourselves with the victims of crime, rather than with the criminals themselves.

Well, I have a small farm with a few horses and I can tell you what that is: horse shit.

If a prisoner can't live out his sentence with some personal integrity, if he can't feel that he has some individual worth, if he is denied the chance to display his particular individuality, what hope does he have of being released to society as a rehabilitated person?

The dangers of depression and dehumanization in confinement are well known to penitentiary people and yet, very often, little is done about it. Certainly conditions have been improved with the establishment of medium and minimum security institutions. But what about maximum security centres?

Maximum security buildings fill a need, but in rehabilitative terms physical surroundings mean little. What is considerably more fundamental is the prisoner's milieu – social, emotional and communal.

Maximum security, as we know it in our institutions, tends to solidify the inmate subculture as the only real community, thus preventing the inmate from developing a sense of independence and individuality without which rehabilitation is probably an unattainable goal.

It is a widely accepted belief that life inside the walls is a jungle-like existence in which the strong prey on the weak, and I'm afraid there is more fact than myth there. In any event, it's virtually impossible to pursue an adequate correctional program with any reasonable hope of success in such circumstances. These conditions tend to create situations in which order and security are jeopardized and insurrection and revolt become real threats.

The situation at K.P. had been aggravated over the years prior to the riot by a steady curtailment of various privileges and inmate programs, ordered reportedly in the interests of promoting security. The result of this approach was a kind of maximum security psychosis which made order and security impossible to maintain.

The inquiry commission was shocked to discover that prior to the riot, inmates at K.P. were obliged to spend at least sixteen hours a day locked in virtual isolation in their cells. There they were free only to sleep, read, write authorized letters and engage in one hobbycraft (provided they had received permission). It wasn't surprising that in these circumstances, many inmates spent their time brooding.

The commission was shocked again when it examined the regimentation in effect even within the confines of the cells themselves. Inmates were restricted in their efforts to decorate their quarters, for example. Any personal item, book, clothing, musical instrument or memento no matter how insignificant, for which a prisoner did not have an institution-issued licence, was contraband and subject to seizure. Individuality in clothing and haircuts was regulated to achieve maximum conformity.

Concerning these points, the inquiry report had this to say:

"The cumulative effect of these factors is first to increase the likelihood that the inmate will become highly institutionalized and submissive to the inmate subculture, and second, to impair seriously his ability to adjust to the community at large on release. Such a regime does a real injustice to a human being and is destructive of whatever humanity may be within him."

There were reasons for the riot at Kingston Penitentiary. There are always reasons, whenever and wherever trouble breaks out. The point is we have to find them and correct them.

**CHAPTER 4**

# Millhaven: The Super-Maximum Prison

The inmates are in the recreation yard, doing what they always do on their afternoon breaks – walking, jogging, shooting the breeze with old buddies, uttering the occasional high-pitched catcall for no reason other than to blow off steam. From the tower, a guard observes the scene. Forty men by actual count. Tall ones, short ones, skinny ones (due to balanced, nutritional meals and controlled intake of food, there are no fat men in prison), old ones, young ones. But in prison denims everybody looks the same.

At the sound of a bell, the men file into the workshop buildings. Moments later, the guards rush into the yard. There's a small heap of denim at the far end. It's Buddy. Somebody ran a *shiv* into him. There is blood on his shirt. He's quite dead.

Some irate editorialist wants an answer. Murder, he pontificates, can't be ignored. Even murder of an inmate. Penal officials agree. They want answers, too. There is an investigation – but no answers. The only witnesses to Buddy's murder were among the forty men in the yard and they have *dummied up* which, in prison parlance, means they aren't talking.

Buddy, we learned later through the grapevine (that clandestine, yet remarkably reliable communications network that collects and reports all kinds of inmate news) had gotten into somebody's bad books by reneging on some old gambling debt. And that day in the yard, he had received his come-uppance. It was what the underworld might have called a settling of accounts.

Have we lost control of our inmates? What goes on in our federal lockups? People put those questions to me all the time. I try to avoid long, heavy discussions about the penal system. No, I answer, we haven't lost control, despite the emergence of a penal philosophy that admits inmates have rights. But on the second question, I pause. What goes on? Well, sometimes, plenty.

Somebody's got the jitters and is apt to pounce on the first person who bugs him. Somebody else thinks there's a contract out on his life and wants to go into segregation to be safe. Who kids about things like that? Get him out of circulation. Pronto. Still another inmate figures life isn't worth the effort. He's been sitting in his cell, brooding. Now his arm is slashed up to here.

Sometimes, you feel the jitters in the joint. Don't ask me to put the feeling into words. It's just there. You feel it in your bones. And the longer you hang around the prisons, the more sensitive you become.

Back in the 1930's when I was a medical student at Queen's University, I decided that I would never be one of those doctors who saw people on certain afternoons and evenings. I would, I decided, be available at all hours. I was to realize that wish. Fortunately, both my first wife, Madeline, who died in 1961, and my present wife, Jane, were able to accept my work habits without much complaint. But when there is trouble in an institution, there is a certain undisguised tension at home.

"George," Jane will say sometimes when I'm answering a special call, "take care." And there will be something in her voice that tells me she is, well, perhaps not exactly scared, but a little worried.

I just shrug when that happens. What have I got to worry about, I always say. The inmates don't think of me as a custodial person. I'm an outsider to them, someone with whom they can talk if they want to get something off their chests.

And yet, I walk into the pen some days and there's that certain something in the air. A kind of sullenness. I can't put my finger on it but the guards have caught a whiff of it too, and they're a little apprehensive.

"Hey, Doc," somebody calls out as I walk through the dome, "how ya doin'?"

The question is friendly but a little later I walk past a group of chatting inmates, on a work break, and suddenly they stop talking. There isn't a friendly grin among them. I have interrupted them and realize I'm on alien territory.

I have never worried about my safety in the penitentiary and I am not about to start now. But I have to admit that, no matter how you look at it, prison is a goddamned dangerous place.

Just when I think that things have quieted down, I run into an agitated, yelping old pro like Mike. "The way he feels today, he could beat the hell out of the Sundance Kid," an officer says. And he looks as though he sure enough could.

Mike is a holdup man but is kind of kinky. On this occasion, he has injected some of his saliva into one of his leg muscles, using a syringe that somebody got for him from...well, who knows where? You can get almost anything in prison if you have the right connections.

Saliva contains certain enzymes that break down food, so if you inject it into the muscle of a leg, for example, it follows its normal destructive process. It eats away at the flesh and you can lose your leg.

"That was a stupid fucking thing to do," an inmate said when Mike told him what he had done. It was a pretty fair conclusion because the saliva had produced a thrombosis and he was in great pain.

"Who cares if I lose a leg?"

Mike was yelling at the top of his voice as they took him into the prison hospital.

"You know what? I don't need two legs. I got $30,000 stashed away in Edmonton."

As it turned out, he didn't lose his leg. As for the $30,000, he never mentioned it again and nobody thought to question him about it.

* * *

Sociologists tell us that ethnic groups in large metropolitan areas develop special sets of characteristics in order to maintain their identification in the face of absorption into the larger, more powerful culture.

Like the ethnics of the free world, inmates develop prison-oriented characteristics. They also support a subcultural society that retains its own codes, values, habits and interests. The prison culture is composed exclusively of inmates who identify with each other and who have strong group loyalties and a very strict code of behavior.

Treason in free society is perhaps the greatest of all crimes. In prison, it has a similar value. An informer, or *stool pigeon*, is the most despicable of all inmates and completely rejected by all levels of the culture. His isolation and punishment are more severe than in the free culture outside.

The prison subculture has several social levels. The aggressives, the bank robbers and assault types, form the core of the inmate society. In this core, decisions are taken to counteract whatever injustice has been done. Here, trouble is fermented, retaliation directed and the tone of the inmate world developed. A larger circle of thieves, robbers and the like stands immediate to the core. A larger and less integrated circle forms the periphery. It is made up of offenders with the least respect in the inmate hierarchy: the child molester, the incestuous offender, arsonists and all other offenders whose crime contains a large emotional component.

The prison society operates its own civilization in a careful and observant way. A continuous battle is waged against the major culture, which includes custodial officers, keepers and wardens. Severe rules will evoke strong reaction from the inmate culture. Lax and poorly enforced regulations excite the subculture into seeking more privileges and demanding more rights.

It's a continuous battle between authority and inmate and each side attempts to exploit the other's weaknesses. Certain inmates are always on the lookout for a guard who will bring a bottle of real booze into the institution for a fee. They don't mind paying twenty dollars in street money for a five-dollar mickey. Not many guards will do this but it would be naive to think there were none. In fairness to the officers, it has to be conceded that occasionally one of their number will agree to bring a pack of cards, or something innocent like that, into the prison out of misplaced sympathy. He then leaves himself open to becoming a tool of the subculture. He is not respected for what he has done and is used in future like a messenger boy.

On the other side of the picture, an inmate may be given certain privileges by the custodial staff with the understanding that he will pass on relevant information on prison activities. Such an inmate, of course, doesn't endear himself to his society.

The inmate culture abhors weakness and indecision on the part of custodial forces. Oddly enough, it expects these forces to live up to their promises. It agrees with discipline if it is fair and specific. Vacillation is a sign of weakness. Unreasonable restrictions are handled carefully. Explanations are asked for. If they are not given, there may be a slowdown in some of the shops, or a small fire may break out somewhere.

Inmates dislike mediocrity. An escape attempt draws respect – but only if it is successful. One inmate who escaped hid in a rhubarb patch close to the institution and was nabbed by a search party soon after his escape. He immediately lost the respect of his fellows and now carries the nickname, "Rhubarb."

The inmate and custodial cultures have a radar-like awareness of each other's activities. It it always a mystery to custodial people when inmates know all about projected moves and new appointments long before officials have released the information. Inmates are also good at learning about planned cell searches. How they get this information is also a mystery to the staff but the inmates start moving their contraband from their cells to another area of the prison, one that has just recently been frisked and is not likely to be searched again.

Contraband may include a wide variety of things – a *shiv* or two, yeast for a future alcohol binge, hoarded food. One inmate recently managed to accumulate and stash away an entire bushel of "Cheerios." Custodial people, on the other hand, also have a sixth sense about the inmate population. They can detect the odors of fermentation and locate a still. They know that if there are fruit flies hovering over an area not normally reserved for food, someone's got a fruit brew in the making. They know that when the mess hall is quiet over a period of days that trouble is brewing. Quiet inmates are often sullen inmates.

Between the two cultures, there exist three neutral areas: the padre, the psychiatrist, and the classification department. These three are excluded by the inmate in his stand against authority. All these areas are bargaining zones, where a voice, a message, can be passed on. Sometimes, inmates come to see me to try to gain special privileges. They do the same with clerical people. Often, they are manipulators. Just as often, they are not. A visit to the padre, or to the psychiatrist, for many, is simply talk therapy, a period in which they can get something off their chests without fear of incrimination.

It's a strange world and the people in it can be mighty strange at times – but let's look at this society of outcasts from another angle. I don't mean in terms of rehabilitation, or politics, or an argument about whether a penitentiary should be located in this area or that. Let us think rather of the man himself. Let's think of him on Saturday night when we're entertaining our friends, or on Sunday afternoon when we're with our children. Let's think of him at six o'clock in the morning when the closeness of another being is so comforting.

His incarceration is his penalty for breaking our social rules and he deserves his lot, and perhaps more. But let us remember that all inmates are not kingpins in the captive society. They are not all ringleaders and trouble-makers. They are not all vicious. They don't all carry knives and they are not all perverted. Inmates can, and very often do, believe in goodness, loyalty and kindness. Some of those people behind bars are kinder and more loyal to their friends than a good many people I know on the outside who have never been in trouble with the law. Inmates don't always have the same set of rules as do people in the free society, but then their rules are based on the sum total of their experiences.

Inmates suffer loneliness, rejection, anguish, hate – everything, in fact, that free people suffer. But when they have a problem, they can't reach for a telephone and speak to a loved one. They can't patch up a disagreement. They can't attend the funeral of a father, or mother. They miss these things, and it is the missing of them that forms the crux of the imprisonment problem.

Man loses more than his freedom when he goes to jail. He trades his name for a number that will be imprinted on everything for the duration of his stay behind bars, wears clothing that is identical to everyone else's, and voids, showers, eats, sleeps, and works at specific, pre-set times. He is robbed of his privacy, his individuality and his possessions. His every act is monitorized – and monotonized.

Prisoners have no individuality. What would any of us do if we were not identified as individuals? The problem is an overwhelming one for the inmate and he will try to be different in one way or another. He may seek a prison position where he has a different uniform. He will cherish his number because it denotes his own particular date of admission (although he also hates his number because it replaces his name). He will try to acquire anything that sets him apart from others. A Red Cross badge for giving several transfusions is an important item. He will try to get a different belt, or he might grow a moustache. He may talk big to get attention from the more gullible inmates. He just hates being a nothing. He wants to be different, to mean something. He may tattoo himself so that the rest of the tribe will know he bears the marks of a kind of great warrior – marks of identification.

A person's success in the eyes of the outside world depends on the scope of his material goods, whether they be apartments, real estate or motor cars. A person with no possessions is an unimportant person. There is an instinctual desire in people to possess, often to possess things different from those of others. In penitentiary, this instinctual drive is stifled before it begins. The inmate is allowed none of his own material possessions. A ring or wristwatch may be allowed but even then there must be some significant reason. Imagine the possession-hungry man, seeking desperately for something to possess, something he can call his own. Frustration is an obvious result.

An inmate is given a canteen allowance for the purchase of cigarette makings, chocolate bars and gum, items which gain a greater intrinsic value because they are possessed. The chocolate bars may be saved for weeks, to be used at a particular time and in particularly important circumstances. They and the cigarette makings become currency items.

Trading is a direct offshoot of possessing. Trading, in the prison world, is the ancient barter economy, and bartering outweighs any other activity in importance. Articles of little significance in free society often assume real value in the institution. An old pair of civilian shoes, left behind by a department officer, not long ago brought thirty-seven packages of cigarettes on the barter market. Petit-point, made in the hobby department, is an active item. Classical subjects like the famous Blue Boy easily bring forty packs of cigarettes at the start, and they are sold over and over again, each time at a higher price.

The custodial forces frown on all of this because bartering and possessing become tools of power. They frown even more on the presence of actual street money, which is entirely taboo behind the walls. However, real money does get in from time to time and it is really valuable. The Canadian dollar may be worth only eighty-odd cents on the U.S. money market but at K.P., it's worth an even ten dollars and it will buy ten dollars' worth of prison goods. The possessive drive varies in intensity but becomes stronger in proportion to the length of the sentence. The less there is to look forward to in terms of release, the greater the importance of possessiveness. The men who hold power in the inmate society are the possessors.

Loss of privacy is a frequently-heard complaint of the new inmate. He resents lining up for meals and walking semi-nude from cell to shower. He resents intrusion into a previously private experience – his toilet. He may become angry because someone else's radio isn't turned down on his specific request. He resents his own lack of importance.

An inmate soon re-establishes his private needs, however, and a new privacy takes shape. His cell becomes the territory of privacy, containing all of his private affairs. The cell is as specifically a projection of his personality as his conversation or his smile. The inmate code says you must never open someone's cell door, even if that someone is your best friend. You must never invade an inmate's privacy until properly invited. Privacy becomes established on a wider scale when a group relationship develops between inmates. This collective privacy is self-reinforcing and keeps other inmates out of the private relationships.

Loss of communication is another problem. Man in free society communicates his likes and dislikes, frets about a newspaper editorial, laughs at the comics, writes letters, converses with emotional significance about many things, reads paperbacks of his choice and is in a continuous, sensitive state of communication, both ingoing and outgoing, with his total world.

In prison, this instinctive force is muted. Verbal communication is frowned upon when the conversation involves more than two people. The philosophy is that while the seeds of contentment rest in communication, the seeds of rebellion are sown in a meeting of minds. Individuals seen talking quietly together are immediately suspect.

General conversation in prison is of a perfunctory nature. Perhaps forty sentences will make up the average inmate's conversation for a day. Speech, too, regresses to a stock slang level of prison nomenclature. A *fish* is a new inmate, a *deuce* is a two-year term, a *diddler* is a person who plays sexually with children, a *merchant* is an inmate who buys and sells things, a *hack* is a female guard and a *screw* is a male guard.

Written communication alters when an individual enters prison. This contact with the outside world is controlled. Each inmate has an approved list of correspondents to whom he may write. His mail is censored, both outgoing and incoming. The inmate knows his communications are never private and infers that the censor is interested in his personal business. Some inmates devise methods of getting letters out illegally. This is called *kiting*. If detected, they are disciplined by loss of privilege. Some prisoners literally write reams and reams of letters, as if some frantic lifeline had to be maintained. Others cease writing altogether after a few weeks of being inside.

Verbal communication with the outside world through the telephone is an extremely precious adventure. A phone call may awaken valued sentiments, may explode controlled emotions and may, in some cases, be as unreal as a Martian visit. But to be permitted to make a call is forever remembered and valued.

**CHAPTER 5**

# Hostage-taking: A Sucker's Game

They go around like zombies, trapped in a world of steel bars and long gray corridors. As new penitentiary inmates, they aren't sure what's happening. Later, they will be able to identify those first stunning experiences as "admission fog."

In a way, it's like living in a psychological cemetery.

The crime, the trial and the intermediate jail sentence pale in contrast to the final loss of freedom, the impersonality of number and cell. The new inmate, starting a long sentence, goes into a state of complete indifference to his prison situation and past emotional experience.

**Admission Fog**

This is not true mental regression. There is no evidence of dependency. In a kind of shock reaction, the inmate simply represses all meaningful emotions, lives in a world of mechanical functions, has little desire to think of yesterday, and even less desire to think of tomorrow. His symptoms during this period of disorientation are seclusiveness, lack of interest in conversation, bland obedience to rules and a disinclination to physical activity, whether work or exercise.

It would seem that the individual's protective mechanisms have pulled a blanket over his senses, his awareness and his reactions. The condition is self-relieving over the months with an increase in the person's sociability and a renewed concern for future plans.

Admission fog is one of several emotional and mental experiences that produce striking alterations in behavior among inmates. These are typified by aberrant emotional phenomena which are not seen in the consulting rooms of free society.

Such phenomena has become less commonplace in penitentiaries in recent years due to the new, more humane approach to imprisonment. Increased privileges and work opportunities and the generally more permissive inmate society have lessened the impact of incarceration. However, the syndromes likely will exist for as long as we keep people behind bars and under lock and key.

The basis of these psychiatric syndromes is the fact that practically all inmates have severe disturbances in their social value systems. Their characteristics include strong elements of hate, aggression, frustration, selfishness, loneliness, hopelessness and intolerance. Each reflects conclusive evidence of repeated childhood disappointments with reactive rebelliousness to hide the hurt, and finally an emotional isolation from the longed-for protective love and warmth. The prison culture reflects these forces with frequent evidence of behavioral types which are more primitive than psychiatric, more protective than purposeful, and more pathological than planned.

Inmates go through a variety of psychiatric conditions during their stays behind bars and some of them can be very serious.

Admission fog is often followed by a condition known as "coasting." This is a psychological state of acceptance of the status quo of prison existence, with rejection of all emotional values in the outside world. This protective, self-imposed isolation compels the inmate to refuse visitors and to stop writing letters and limits his interest to immediate prison adjustments. Contact with the outside world can produce severe anxiety, irradiated hostility, tension, sleeplessness and even suicidal impulses. The condition slowly disappears as the inmate's friends and relatives in the outside world reassure him of his importance to them.

Some of the other conditions may be summarized as follows:

**Lockup Request**

This unusual request for isolation within isolation, also known as a "crisis request" is a phenomenon of the prison subculture, indicating that the inmate no longer can handle his prison experiences. After months of precarious adjustment, he is torn by explosive, destructive forces which can take the form of an attack on an inmate, an officer, or even himself. He requests to be locked up to re-establish his self-control. In this way, he withdraws into a world of mental inactivity with complete isolation from all physical and emotional experiences.

This condition is usually indicative of unresolved inmate problems but may also reflect a developing psychopathology, that is, a potential mental illnes. Physical retreat into solitude is therapeutic in itself, however, and allows the inmate to sort out his problems. Counselling and psychotheraphy may be helpful during this period of crisis.

**Isolation Sickness**

Prolonged solitary confinement, protective or punitive, may produce a massive psychological reaction due to deprivation of accustomed sensory input.This sickness produces reactions identical to those of victims of brainwashing techniques used by the Nazis during the Second World War and has been simulated by psychologists in experimental situations. This is a psychotic reaction, characterized by hallucinations and delusions, produced by prolonged physical isolation and inactivity in completely segregated areas.

Medical assessment of the isolated offender will record increased motor activity to supply kinaesthetic sensation, and auditory hallucinations to compensate for the lack of sound stimuli. The inmate may even talk loudly to himself to increase his sensory experiences. Reality may be altered by misinterpretation of stimuli to produce suspicions and feelings of persecution.

Violent aggression or intense suicidal drives may be the inmate's response to his terrifying mental state. Prompt removal of the individual from isolation and judicious use of sedation and appropriate psychological stimulation will reverse the situation.

**Stir Crazy**

This is a term that has been bandied about over a great many years, often in a humorous vein. In technical fact, it classifies the inmate's protective regression to a childish state of silly, petulant behavior. It is symptomized by forgetfulness, difficulty in concentration, inept conversation, inattention to work and a disregard to future planning.

Inmates and officers are treated with casual, almost playful indifference. The inmate's preoccupation with his date of release may assume obsessive proportions. Impulsive rages are precipitated by minor irritations. The condition improves under supportive counselling and intensified athletic work.

**Slashing Syndrome**

Self-mutilation is a mute expression of pent-up anger, resentment and frustration. The original problem is submerged in favor of a more immediate attention-getting device, and a sharp instrument becomes the inmate's passport to the protective atmosphere of medical care.

Suicide is seldom the prime intent in self-mutilation, although serious slashing has resulted, in numerous instances, in extensive cuts and lacerations, requiring suturing and transfusion. Continued frustration may then cause the inmate to reopen his wounds and purposely contaminate them, thus necessitating further medical attention.

Slashing can become epidemic in an institution, if appropriate disciplinary measures are not taken. The slasher's actions usually are planned and purposeful. They are designed to solve an immediate problem, and they are also an indignant expression of hostility toward the custodial forces. There is a secondary emotional gain for the slasher in the sympathy and attention he generates among a previously uninterested inmate population. Attention must be directed to solving the basic problem through counselling or psychiatric treatment.

**The Phantom Female**

Men's preference for male company is not a disturbing problem.

Meaningful emotional relationships between men are seen in warfare, sports and family loyalties. But such conditions in the prison subculture carry additional sexual components. A mature male may find a female surrogate figure in a young male inmate. Endearments and gift-sending identify the relationship as a phantom heterosexual affair. The young male with his adolescent smile, his unsophisticated manners, his soft skin and esthetic proportions, embodies the female. The relationship assumes a protective, benevolent role. The young inmate inevitably surrenders either voluntarily or forcibly to the seductive desires of the older male. Upon release, the older man drops his façade and prepares himself for his more true desires. The younger man, too, grows out of his romance to become a prison-wise member of the inmate society. There are no intrinsic homosexual characteristics in either participant. It has simply been a "marriage of convenience." There is no "hangover" when the parties return to the society of conformers.

**Homosexual Panic**

This condition occurs when a man fears he may be contemplating a homosexual act, strongly against what he thought was his nature. The guilt of sexual awareness, combined with a desire to show affection to another, is magnified by the fear of submitting to homosexual temptation. Degrees of panic may result, with marked fears, senseless physical activities, and ideas of persecution. In final desperation, suicide may be attempted. Such cases require immediate psychiatric attention in a controlled, non-threatening environment.

**Gate Fever**

Awareness that their release and return to free society is imminent stirs up marked anxiety in many inmates. This anxiety, with irritability and sleeplessness, develops three to four weeks before release and bears directly on the inmate's knowledge that he is poorly equipped to adjust to the competitive, aggressive society outside. The problems of planning one's life, facing unresolved problems and being responsible for one's actions may be so overwhelming that the individual begins to anticipate an early return to his prison existence long before he is actually released.

These are the psychiatric syndromes of institutional life and can be proven clinically in any prison environment. There are almost identical observations to be found in reports on servicemen held as prisoners of war between 1939 and 1945. The question is this: If an individual develops fog, coasting and gate fever in the prison culture, will he not face similar conditions as a free man? The answer is that a man's reactions to life situations are not likely to change.

Inmates released after years of imprisonment describe a pronounced state of stupor and confusion on release. The condition lasts six to eight months, exactly like admission fog. The barrage of sensory experiences is likely to push these people even deeper into the fog state. They also report a frequent loss of ambition for jobs and general security. Coasting is reflected in a prevalent lack of animation among ex-inmates. Finally, the old pre-release fever is often re-lived in a pre-employment period of doubt and anxiety. Psychiatric syndromes thus continue to obstruct life for those released.

Released inmates, regardless of their previous offences, have to overcome a great many obstacles if they are to be reinstated into the outside world. The problem, of course, is that free society will not really allow them to be treated as free people. In its vindictive way, society wants to perpetuate the felonic image of inmates as cold, despicable, dangerous people.

But are they really all that despicable and dangerous? The answer has to be that some are – and some are not. Most, in fact, are not. Practically every known variety of criminal has passed through the old stone fortress of Kingston Penitentiary at one time or another during the more than twenty years of my association with it, and virtually every one of them has sat down across the desk from me and told me his story.

It has been good therapy on both sides of the desk. I think some of the inmates have learned something from me. I know I've learned a lot from them.

**CHAPTER 6**

# The Criminal Personality

The oldtimers affectionately named their little village on the shores of Lake Ontario, about fifteen miles west of Kingston, Millhaven, because a mill stood there and because it was a safe haven for ships in stormy weather. Some of the country's toughest criminals know it today as the site of Canada's super maximum security penitentiary, Millhaven Institution. They call it, unaffectionately, "The Mill" where the chaff is beaten out of your goddamned head.

Inmates will tell you flatly that anybody who thinks he's safe behind bars ain't been to Millhaven. "Like man," a black inmate I know says, "you gotta have three pairs of eyes when you're in there. You got one pair up front, one pair at the back of your head and another pair in your pocket in case you need replacements."

The Dirty Dozen will tell you how tough that place is. As ringleaders of the K.P. riot, transferred to Millhaven, they got an initiation they wouldn't soon forget. Who, they asked one another, gets a reception like that when they go into prison, especially on a transfer?

Custodial officers stood in an inside passageway known as P Corridor, through which the new arrivals would have to pass as they entered the institution. The officers, armed with riot sticks, stood eight feet apart, thus assuring that no inmate passing through would be out of range of them. Then whack, whack, whack...

It was the old game of "running the gauntlet" and one inmate quipped later, "They're making it as hard to get into this joint as to get out."

Things aren't as bad at Millhaven as some inmates would have you believe but as the institution's psychiatrist (an extension of my activities at the Regional Psychiatric Centre) I have to admit that life there has its uneasy moments. Protests, sit-downs, slow-downs, small fires, slashings, hostage incidents – there is usually enough doing, or in the making, to keep the staff on its toes.

"Sixty goddamned riots in five years," Don Flynn says. "That's what they had out there before I left."

I correct him. "They weren't riots," I explain.

"What the hell do you call them then?"

"Disturbances, Don. Not riots."

Like I say, when trouble breaks out, there has to be a reason, even if it isn't bobbing around on the surface for everyone to see. Finding the source of the trouble that erupted at Millhaven in the summer of 1980, however, wasn't easy.

Why would four inmates, three of whom had less than a year of their sentences to serve and one who was eligible for release in 1982, be stupid enough to get involved in a hostage-taking incident? Why would they take two prison shop instructors hostage in such an obviously futile attempt to win transfers to a British Columbia penitentiary?

Penal officials were stumped. It just didn't make sense for the four to risk longer sentences and possible death in a shootout with guards to press demands for transfers. (Hostage-takers usually get about three years on charges of forcible confinement and assault.)

The final outcome of the incident was predictable. The hostages were released unharmed after eleven hours and their captors were sent to Millhaven's Special Handling Unit, a kind of prison-within-a-prison, set up in the 1970's to handle the real hardcore types.

It was not until early 1981 that the real story of the hostage-taking began to unravel. The man who told the story was a recently-released inmate named Brian who claimed the four men had taken their desperate action out of sheer fear for their lives. They thought – in fact, they were convinced – that if they stayed at Millhaven, they would be murdered.

Brian didn't mince words. He said a climate of violence existed in the prison and charged that the administration was responsible for it. The administration, naturally enough, denied the charge.

The trouble actually started back in the Spring of 1980 when a group of inmates arrived at Millhaven on a routine transfer from the Pacific region. Such transfers are involuntary and often organized as a means of scattering troublemakers. Inmates are against these transfers and as former chairman of the Odyssey Group, an inmates' rights organization, Brian became involved.

He said the new batch of westerners were angry and frustrated. They didn't like Millhaven, they didn't like Millhaven's programs and furthermore, they didn't particularly like Millhaven's residents. It was a bad start.

Trouble broke out sporadically. Then one day, a group of inmates beat up four of the newcomers in the recreation yard. It was all done quietly. Well, relatively speaking. Not a word was exchanged. The attackers, armed with baseball bats and knives, beat their victims and chased them around the yard. Guards brought the incident to an end when they started shooting over the inmates' heads. The four injured men were taken to hospital and later assigned to segregation cells for their protection.

As many as twenty men may have been in the attacking party but only six were identified. They, too, were immediately placed in segregation. No charges were laid because, in keeping with normal inmate practice, no one would testify against them. An angry Ron, however, said the institution had set the stage for the subsequent hostage-taking by not laying charges.

"For the rest of the guys from out west, it meant that the Millhaven inmates had a license to beat them up," he told a Kingston Whig-Standard reporter. "The four guys who took the hostages were terrified. They figured they were going to get it and they were scared. Real scared. Like, they had to get out and it wasn't because they didn't like the steak sauce."

Knowing that somebody is out to get you in prison is probably the most frightening experience an inmate can have. There is really only one place you can hide: in a segregation cell. But some time or other, you're going to have to come out.

In fact, only three of the four hostage-takers were from the west. Jack, 23, serving eight years and eight months for manslaughter, was from Edmonton; Charlie, 41, serving five years for narcotics trafficking, was from Armstrong, B.C.; and George, 34, serving three years for robbery, was from Fisher River, Manitoba. The fourth man, Guy, 19, doing four years for theft, attempting to pass a forged document and possession of a dangerous weapon, was from Sarnia, Ontario and had been transferred from Warkworth Institution.

You might have expected Millhaven to quiet down after the hostage-taking incident. It didn't. Brian said that because of past events, new inmates arrived at Millhaven convinced that they had to be tough to survive. This is the way he put it:

"I got scared of guys coming in that don't even shave. Now you got all the punks and riff-raff coming in who are violent because they think it's expected. At one time, you didn't have to be scared of anybody in there. You can't play floor hockey in that place now. People are just terrified."

Millhaven has had some uneasy moments apart from the hostage affair. Inmates staged a sit-down strike on one occasion in protest against an administrative decision to lock up two men for drinking. Later, an inmate in the Special Handling Unit set fire to his cell. A fight broke out between prisoners and the guards used tear gas to get them back to their cells. Three inmates were hurt in the fighting.

But that wasn't all.

On October 13, 1980, an inmate named Larry, 23, of Kapuskasing, Ontario, was found stabbed to death in his cell. On October 21, Mark, 32, of Hamilton, was stabbed to death in his cell. On November 24, authorities chalked up another murder: that of Paul, 30, of Brantford, Ontario. On January 31, 1981, guards walked into the cell of Fred, 20, and found him dead of a knife wound.

Bob, of New Westminster, B.C. was luckier. He received serious stab wounds while doing time in the Special Handling Unit in October, 1980, but survived.

Millhaven officials had no formal explanations for the troubles that plagued the institution. Brian did. He blamed them largely on involuntary transfers. It was frustration, he said. The inmates didn't want to be transferred and they refused to fit into prison programs.

There's always a reason.

**CHAPTER 7**

# The Prison Subculture

For an inmate, taking hostages is a sucker's game. He can't win. The odds are stacked too heavily against him. To start with, he can be sure of serving extra years for his trouble. Worse, he might get picked off by one of those dead-eye guys with the rifles. There are some really top-notch marksmen in those penitentiaries. And some of them think they're doing the world a big favor by getting rid of hostage-takers.

Yet hostage incidents are happening all the time. Why? Basically, holding people captive is the aggressive inmate's way of drawing attention to himself and the problem that's bugging him.

Take Gary, for example.

Gary harbored strong feelings of anxiety and hostility. At twenty-eight, he had served a year of a twenty-year sentence for an armed robbery he said he hadn't committed. I know our prisons are full of people who claim they're serving time for a crime they didn't do, but Gary...well, I'm not in a position to judge him. He maintained that he had been dealt with wrongly, and he was determined to "get back at the system."

In any event, he had grandiose plans for settling the score.

He was going to blow up K.P.'s sewage system, he told me one day. He was going to mix a gallon of the ammonia found in cleaning powders with a gallon of vinegar and pour the solution down the toilets, stuffing great wads of toilet paper into one of the bowls so as to block the effluent pipes and keep the solution from running off. The chemical reaction supposedly would cause explosions in the pipes.

Gary never carried out that plan but on July 31, 1961, he put an even more dramatic plan into operation. He did it with the help of an inmate, Jean, 27, who was doing fifteen years for armed robbery. Jean had been transferred from Montreal's St. Vincent de Paul Penitentiary, where he had made knife attacks on guards and other inmates.

Gary and Jean ambushed five officers and held them hostage in a mezzanine room above the kitchen. The room had windows from which officers normally surveyed activities in the kitchen below. The ambush took place late Friday afternoon, and after I had left my office at K.P. I heard about it when I got home and switched on the six o'clock news. The news item was brief: two inmates were holding five officers at knife-point. There were no other details.

My late first wife, Madeline, and I spent that evening and all the next day glued to the radio. Prison officials had tried to negotiate some sort of truce with Gary but had failed. It was a stalemate. By Sunday morning, I was getting uneasy. A hostage incident that lasts more than twenty-four hours is in a crucial stage. The situation can get so tense that even a small incident might trigger a major reaction. At 2 p.m., the telephone rang. It was Jarvis, the warden, asking me to go to the prison. I wasn't surprised by the call. When things get bad enough behind the walls, you call in the psychiatrist. Actually, in those days, the shrink wasn't viewed as being a very useful person although he was supposed to possess peculiar powers such as hypnosis and the ability to psychoanalyze people merely by talking to them for a few minutes.

Jarvis, a tough, square-jawed, hard-hitter was able to handle men. Normally. Gary and Jean were something else. Gary had yelled down from the mezzanine window earlier that if any attempt was made to rush him, or if tear gas was used, he would behead each of the guards he held hostage and throw the heads, one by one, down to the kitchen floor below.

Later, Jarvis said, Gary called out, "I don't know what you guys got in mind but if any bastards are thinking of coming up here, this is a warning. I'll take their eyes out (the hostages' eyes) and I'll throw them down there one by one, and then they'll be looking at you for a long time, them dead eyes."

Sometimes I think I've got guts. Other times, I just think I'm a damned fool. I don't know which it was, guts or idiocy, that Sunday afternoon at K.P. but I agreed to go up and talk to Gary. Penitentiary officials had made no headway with him. A Justice Department representative named James Macaulay, sent down from Ottawa to negotiate an end to the crisis, had gotten nowhere and, as a matter of fact, was sitting up on the mezzanize with him, a virtual hostage himself. I was a kind of last resort, I guess. Anyway, Gary agreed to see me. We weren't exactly strangers at this point. An American with no family or friends nearby, he had requested consultations with me some months earlier because he was very upset about his sentence. It seems like a strange thing to say but I rather liked Gary in spite of his persecution complex and hostile nature.

I climbed the steps to the mezzanine alone and Gary met me at the door. "Hello, Doc," he said, casually, as though he was greeting a friend at home.

"Hello, Gary, what's going on here?" I said. What a dumb question. The five hostages were lying face down on the floor, tied with strong meat-binding string. Trussed together in a series, they were attached like fish on a length of cord. In the centre of the room, Macaulay sat motionless, his pinstripe suit and briefcase looking very strange in these surroundings. Behind me was Gary's French cohort, Jean. Feeling menaced, I demanded, "What's that guy doing behind me?"

Gary made a sign and Jean came around in front of me.

There are two major ground rules in hostage-taking. First, you make sure that the hostages are released unharmed. Second, you look for a way out of your predicament without losing face. I tried to impress these two points on Gary.

"Is there some place we can talk privately?" I asked, thinking he might talk more openly if he knew the conversation was just between ourselves. The only private place was the toilet – and there we talked. For the longest fifteen minutes of my life.

"I didn't come here with a deal," I said at the outset. "I've got no authority to promise anybody anything but if I say I'm going to try to help you, you know I will. I think you know that I always do my best for the guys in the joint." This was no bullshit. I always did.

"I tried to talk to the guy from Ottawa," Gary said. "But he doesn't know anything about anything. He has the authority to negotiate but how the fuck can he negotiate emotions? I mean I'm not wanting to change my fucking cell, or something."

His facial muscles were frozen as he talked. "Sure, I was a pretty lousy kid. I was a pretty fucking erratic teenager. But Jesus, I got no business being here. That was a bum sentence. Every time I think of it, I get furious."

I interrupted to ask if he were armed. He rolled up his shirt sleeve to show a straight razor, strapped neatly on the inside of his forearm with cellophane. I told him the most important thing in my mind at that moment was how he was going to get out of a very awkward situation.

"Those guys on the floor out there," I said. "They're going to get angry. Eighteen hours with their faces on the floor is no picnic. If they all decide to get up together, you're in trouble. Their feet are tied but they can move and if they come down on you, they'll trample you to death. That little knife of yours can't handle a thousand pounds of angry bodies."

Gary was a man of logic. I knew he was smart enough to realize when a situation was untenable. "Look at it this way," I said. "If they rush this place and one officer is injured, you aren't going to survive.

You'll be a very dead Gary and your French friend will be very dead, and so there'll be a dead Frenchman, a dead American, a dead government man and" – I gulped as I contemplated the possibility–"a dead psychiatrist. So, how do we get out of this? Tell me what you want and I'll try to arrange it for you."

He thought for a long moment and then he said, "I want to phone my people. I want to phone my mother in the States. If I can phone her, I think it'll be all right."

He had taken five hostages, held them for almost two full days and risked getting himself shot full of holes. All for one telephone call to his mother.

We stepped out of the toilet into the main room where Jean was guarding the hostages. Gary beckoned him over. "The doc says we better blow this thing," he announced. Jean seemed relieved. The three of us then walked out the door and down the stairs to the kitchen. The steps were like those you find on shipboard, steep with narrow treads, and we all descended cautiously. If someone had slipped, God knows what might have happened. The place was that tense.

The passageway through the kitchen was lined on one side by guards, on the other by kitchen helpers. There were so many people there, it looked like the finish line of a road race. Nobody said anything and I was praying. If one of those big meat cleavers, knives or potato mashers fell from a hook, we were goners. Any sudden noise and the whole goddamned place would have exploded.

I led the way, Gary followed and Jean brought up the rear. Jean left us in the kitchen, surrendering meekly to guards, and Gary and I proceeded to my office in an adjoining building. There I advised the duty officer that we were going to go in and close the door – and not to worry. Everything was all right. I told Gary to sit at my desk and use the telephone to call anyone he wished. It was a big deal. A real big deal. Getting an okay to make a telephone call when you're in prison is like getting an expensive Christmas present.

"When you're through, just rap on the window," I said.

He made his call while I waited outside. Then he tapped on the window and I joined him. He didn't volunteer any information about the call and I didn't ask any questions. "I'm going home, Gary," I said, "and I think you'd better wrap this thing up."

He nodded weakly. The tension and the long hours of sleeplessness were taking their toll. "You bet, Doc," he said finally. There was a small nervous grin on his face. Outside my office, two guards were waiting to return him to his cell.

Gary took the five officers hostage that summer weekend to protest his imprisonment, which he had maintained all along was both unfair and illegal. It was an entirely futile exercise because there is nothing the administration of a prison can do about the sentence of a court. Fortunately, he had someone to talk to – me. And fortunately the incident came to an end before somebody decided to shoot up the place. I don't know where he is today. If he's in jail somewhere on what he thinks is another bum rap, I hope he remembers his adventure in Kingston. If he's lucky, maybe somebody will let him make a phone call before he decides to do something more drastic.

* * *

Planning a hostage-taking is somewhat like planning a bank robbery. You have to think about a great many details. You have to have contingency plans in case something goes wrong. You have to ask yourself beforehand, "if such-and-such a thing happens, what action will I take?" Once you've started the action, it's too late. You can't say, "Oh, I should have done this, or the other thing."

That is the problem with hostage-taking incidents in penitentiaries. Inmates seldom think out the dangerous situations they create. In fact, they seldom have any firm idea of how they are going to handle them at all. And, of course, time is more often on the side of the authorities. They usually can wait out the tiring, weakening captor.

Donald was a case in point. He was what we call an "inadequate" person, one who is emotionally defective, perhaps even a little retarded, and unable to cope with his environment. He had a history of maladjustment as a child, at home and at school. As an adult, he had a difficult time making a living. In 1977, at age twenty-eight, he was in Kingston Penitentiary for assaulting women.

Like so many others, Donald wanted a transfer out of K.P. and one day he decided the way out was by means of a hostage-taking. That day, brandishing a razor, he seized two young women, Cindy Pressé, a psychologist, and Marie Smith, a clerk, who happened to be in Cindy's office. He herded them into a room nearby, closed the door and piled desks and chairs against it so no one could enter.

Donald spent two days locked up with the women, opening the door just slightly to retrieve food and cigarettes that were placed on the floor nearby every few hours. Periodically, he would pick up the phone and call for something or other. Coffee, gum, things like that. It was almost like calling room service in a hotel. I know this all sounds a little strange but the thing you must always remember in situations like these is: keep cool.

I presumed he had told the women that they might be in for a long stay because at one point he announced that his captives needed a change of clothing and asked that the officers please call their homes and make the necessary arrangements. He even provided the telephone numbers.

I wasn't too worried about Donald, the man. He didn't have a history of dangerous behavior, even though he had been convicted of assault. He was not a sex offender and was not known as someone who disliked women. As a matter of fact, he made it clear on the telephone on one occasion that he had no intention of harming his hostages. He had taken them captive, he said, to force the institution to give him a transfer.

What worried me was the time factor. How long was this man capable of functioning without sleep? Sooner or later, he would have to do something about his hostages and if he wanted to sleep, he would have to tie them up. This is the dilemma when there is only one hostage-taker. If he decided to try to keep himself awake, he would be putting his emotional tempo at risk. Chances are, if he didn't sleep, he would become impulsive, unstable, unpredictable and paranoid. Then, of course, he could be dangerous.

Donald began to get the jitters on the second day. The cool, calm voice that spoke to the officers over the telephone earlier was getting raspy. Soon after, he stopped using the telephone. He began shouting, sometimes frantically, through the door. He wanted out. Now.

Then he made his demands. He wanted three bed sheets. He and the hostages would get under them and walk out, the authorities promising safe passage through the main gate and out of the city. (He didn't specify a destination.) It was a unique idea because the sharpshooters wouldn't be able to see their target under the sheets. He also wanted ten thousand dollars in ten-dollar bills.

Unknown to Donald, the institution's six-man Special Weapons and Tactics team, known generally as SWAT and organized expressly to deal with hostage situations, was considering strategy to end the drama.

The SWAT team was equipped with all the latest tools to handle incidents like this one. Among the hardware was an electric saw reputed to be powerful enough to cut through a door like the one in the hostage room in thirty-six seconds flat. Great. But what would Donald be going during those thirty-six seconds? Would he panic and do something desperate?

As it turned out, it wasn't our crack team of experts that saved the day but a plumbing instructor named Pete McConnell, who had known Donald before. It was McConnell who had taken food to the hostage room and delivered fresh clothing for the women. His plan, so unscientific it was almost funny, got the approval of Don Clark, director of the institution, and members of the SWAT team. (The title of Warden was replaced by that of Director in 1973. It reverted to Warden again in 1980).

McConnell placed food just outside the door and crouched down near it. Some minutes later, the door opened slightly and Donald's hand reached out for the dish. McConnell pounced, grabbing his forearm, bending it at the elbow and pinning it to the wall beside the door, fishhook-style. The SWAT team then ripped through one of the walls and took custody of the inmate. True to his word, the hostages had been unharmed.

Sheepishly, Donald went back to his cell, his adventure over, his hopes dashed. Why had he taken such an extreme measure for such a minor issue? He wanted everyone to know about his problem. He would have drawn no attention at all going through regular channels.

* * *

Not all inmates who want to draw attention to their requests resort to hostage-taking. One climbed sixty feet to the top of the big one hundred thousand gallon water tower at Joyceville Institution one summer day in 1978 and announced that he intended to stay there until the authorities gave him a transfer.

I was at the Regional Psychiatric Centre in Kingston when the call came from Reginald Chitty, Joyceville's director. "Can you get me out of a mess?" he wanted to know. I said I'd try.

"This inmate's up on the tower and I want you to go there and talk him into coming down, so that I can talk to him," he said. "He's been up there eighteen hours and we don't know what to do. He's not a dangerous person, so we can't hose him off or shoot him. What do we do?"

Psychiatrists are often thought of–erroneously, I might point out – as magicians. We're supposed to be able to wave a wand and, presto, the problem is solved. Well, it doesn't work that way and besides, I sometimes get turned off by these demonstrators, Clyde included.

"Reg," I said, "leave him there. Pay no attention to him. Eventually, he'll either fall off, or he'll just come down, figuring the exercise isn't worth the effort. In some way, he'll solve his own problem. The trouble with people who start a course of action like this is that they never plan how they're going to end it."

I checked the psychiatric records and found no mention of Clyde. He'd never been a patient, so I had no idea how he functioned. I drove out to Joyceville and, sure enough, there was Clyde, sitting on the very peak of the tank. He had used a tall ladder to reach the top of the tank legs and then had gone up the tank steps.

Chitty filled me in on the details. The officers had gone out on the grounds with loud hailers the moment they had spotted him. Clyde wasn't being very friendly, though. In fact, he was angry. He was tired of being locked up at Joyceville. He wanted a transfer to Warkworth Institution, so he could be near home, and he said he wouldn't come down until he got it. He also threatened to jump if anybody started to climb up the tank.

The security people thought I should try to persuade him to come down. I didn't think so. I had no intention of going up the tower and I had no plans to chat with him through a loud hailer, either. There are limits to what a psychiatrist will do. I asked Chitty to relay a message to Clyde. I was quite prepared to talk things over with him, I said, but it would have to be in a normal, civilized way, in the quiet of an office.

Well, Clyde listened to my message, considered it for a few moments, and came down. Just like that. No fuss, no angry words. We went into a room in the main building and, for about fifteen minutes, I listened. Clyde hadn't wanted that much, really. He was lonely. He missed his family. And he wanted to be where his parents could visit him easily.

Clyde got some additional time tagged on to his sentence – but managed to serve it at Warkworth, where he wanted to be.

**CHAPTER 8**

# Psychiatric Syndromes in Prison

David is twentyish and well-groomed, the kind of nice, clean-cut kid you might find playing basketball at the neighborhood YMCA. He is also the kind of polite, well-mannered boy who might put a bullet in you sometime, given the right set of unhappy circumstances.

David was a big shot out on the street. He held up a loan company, knocked off a supermarket and always carried a sawed-off shotgun around with him even when he wasn't on a job. Just in case somebody decided to give him a bad time. He's in the jug now – and still a big shot. He's known as a trouble-starter, a ringleader, an escape risk. If a riot breaks out, he probably will be one of the leaders. He is what I call a rebel or, to use a more proper psychiatric term, an aggressive personality.

Then there is Wayne. He's about the same age as David and every bit as boy-next-doorish in looks. He doesn't carry a gun and he doesn't like violence. He'd never stick up a bank, for example. He'd starve first. But he'd watch your house, and after seeing you leave, he might break in. They caught him coming out of an apartment building with an Adidas bag full of jewelry not long ago and now he's in a cell on the same range as David. He's a small-time pro, the kind of inmate who prides himself on knowing his way around a prison. He is what I call a *sneak*, or more technically, a passive-aggressive personality, and his kind makes up more than half the population of most penitentiaries.

David and Wayne have certain things in common, and I don't mean their good looks, because this is quite coincidental. Contrary to what many people think, criminals do not fit a particular physical mold. They are not necessarily square-headed, or tough-looking. Some, in fact, are handsome. Others look like businessmen which, of course, they may very well have been. Criminals, in other words, do not have to look like criminals. What David and Wayne have in common is a desire to adhere to the inmate code, which means they pride themselves on never co-operating with the administration. They are also both recidivists, and both stick together in resisting rehabilitation. Beyond that, though, they are not at all alike.

For one thing, David is geared to violence. "This is what I want and I'm going to get it" is his basic philosphy. He is the robber who faces his victim directly and says to his face, "I want your money." In civilian life, he resented being told what to do. In prison, he has the same resentment. He is frequently involved in arguments and believes the only way to resolve them is by physical means. He cannot tolerate controls or limitations in day-to-day life, distrusts advice and, as an expression of hostility, refuses to learn anything. He is destructive on occasion, and unrepentant. Aggressive offenders like him are associated with major crimes such as kidnapping, assault causing bodily harm, assault with intent, wounding with intent, armed robbery, extortion, intimidation, murder, manslaughter and occasionally rape.

Rebels, or aggressives, speak up when confronted. If they don't like something, they say so – directly. They make no secret of their feelings, wishes and needs. David was very straightforward with me in one interview.

"Yeah, I like guns," he said in answer to one of my questions. "I like guns very much."

"Do you carry a gun usually?" I asked. "When you're on the street?"

"I carry a sawed-off shotgun with me all the time."

"How do you do that? Don't those things have big butts?"

"Well, what you do is you cut it down and you wear a benny and you just carry it under your benny."

"A benny?"

"Like, it's an overcoat."

"Like a car coat maybe?"

"Yeah, like a three-quarter benny."

I was curious about why he felt he had to go around armed.

"I just like carrying it. Period."

"What about a toy gun? You could carry one of those. Nobody would have to know it was a toy."

"Naw, I like carrying the real thing. When you got a real gun, people know you mean what you say and they don't fool around."

In prison, David was often in trouble and he admitted it readily.

"I'm a shit disturber. You know what I mean? I mean, like I don't take no for an answer. But if somebody wants to have a riot, well I'm right there with them."

I wanted to know about the inner David. Did he have a capacity for loving people?

"Me, the only thing I've ever loved...that was a gun and a *shiv*. And money. Those things, like that's what I love."

"And people?"

"I don't have no great love for nobody 'cause when I do I'm always the guy who winds up on the wrong end of things."

Wayne presents a different picture. He got what he wanted on the outside by going behind people's backs. He would never face up to someone. He would never confront his victim. That is one thing that is dependable about a sneak-thief. He will never do anything face-to-face and, when imprisoned, will not change his personality orientation. He will never, for instance, tell someone off to his face. Instead, he will be devious because he has been devious all his life. He doesn't possess enough personal strength or drive to adjust satisfactorily to society and satisfy his needs through normally accepted patterns. He doesn't have the personality that allows him, when he wants something, to go out and earn it honestly. He sneaks around, getting his rewards in a more indirect assault on his victims. He belongs to a group of offenders who fill police blotters with break-and-entry charges. He robs houses and stores and steals cars, operating when there is the least danger of meeting the owner.

Wayne had been breaking into houses and motel rooms for about eight years when I talked to him, in fact, since he was about thirteen years of age, and rarely had he ever come into contact with anyone. Now, in prison, he was always surrounded by people, even though they also were criminals. In close quarters like that, arguments are not infrequent.

"Would you ever go up to somebody and say, 'Look, I don't like your face and I'm going to smash you one?' " I asked him.

"Oh, I'm not that kind of guy at all. If I don't like a guy, I just don't *crack* to him (talk to him). I put him on the *dummy* (playing dumb) because I know if I *crack* to the guy, I'm going to get into trouble and I'll probably end up getting the worst beating of my life."

Criminal behavior is a term that has been bandied about a great deal, often in very loose fashion, over the years. My own definition – and one which is certainly open to criticism – is that it is a social value in which behavior is not in harmony with existing social mores and, as a result, is undesirable and actually a social impairment.

I look upon criminal activity as symptomatic of personality conflict, just as a physical symptom can reflect emotional conflict. It is in itself an aberrant expression of neurotic behavior. After many years of study and observation, I believe there is ample proof that, almost without exception, the crime fits the personality of the person who has committed it. When the crime pattern varies, it is because of some altered emotional conflict, or because mental illness has interfered.

But how does one go about defining personality types? Is it possible to categorize personalities so that we can say more than so-and-so is "a nice guy," or that she's "hard to get along with?" Well, yes we can. Psychiatry has succeeded in identifying basic personality types and an understanding of these types is essential if we are to understand the criminal mind.

**The Schizoid Personality**

This type of personality is primarily thoughtful and reflective. The schizoid is more or less controlled and always thinking about his relationship with the world. He is introspective, the kind of person who chooses his own company, rather than the company of a group of people. He is the kind of person who would much rather sit alone and read a book than go to a hockey game with a friend. If he is interested in recreation, he does something by himself, like going for a walk in the woods, or going for a workout in the gymnasium. A schizoid has a personality that is self-contained, not necessarily withdrawn but with a clearly stable system of reference within himself. He does not depend upon other people for emotional nourishment.

**The Cyclothymic Personality**

This is the second basic type of personality. "Cyclo" means a cycle, a turning thing, and "thymic" deals with the mood of the individual. These personalities are subject to dramatic shifts in mood. These are the moody people who feel either wonderfully exhilarated or terribly depressed. They are extremely vulnerable to changes in their immediate environment and respond to them with an inner shift in mood.

The schizoid personality is rigid. This type never reacts much differently from one day to the next. The cyclothymic, on the other hand, has an emotional barometer that is constantly rising or falling because he is continually reacting to the world around him. He is, in fact, the direct opposite of the schizoid, who has his own way of doing things and lets the rest of the world go about its business.

Because the cyclothymic person is always receiving impulses from the outside, he is victimized by his environment. In other words, his reactions to the world are often controlled by the way in which the world affects him. Some cyclothymics have a consistently negative reaction to the world. They are the people who read the morning paper and conclude gloomily that everything is falling apart. Others are optimistic. They are euphoric about experiences and events and, after reading the news, are likely to say, "So what?"

**The Paranoid Personality**

The third basic type is at variance with the world. People in this group are so preoccupied with minding everybody else's business that they can't look after their own. They pat their friends on the back, borrow money from them, and telephone them at night wanting to do

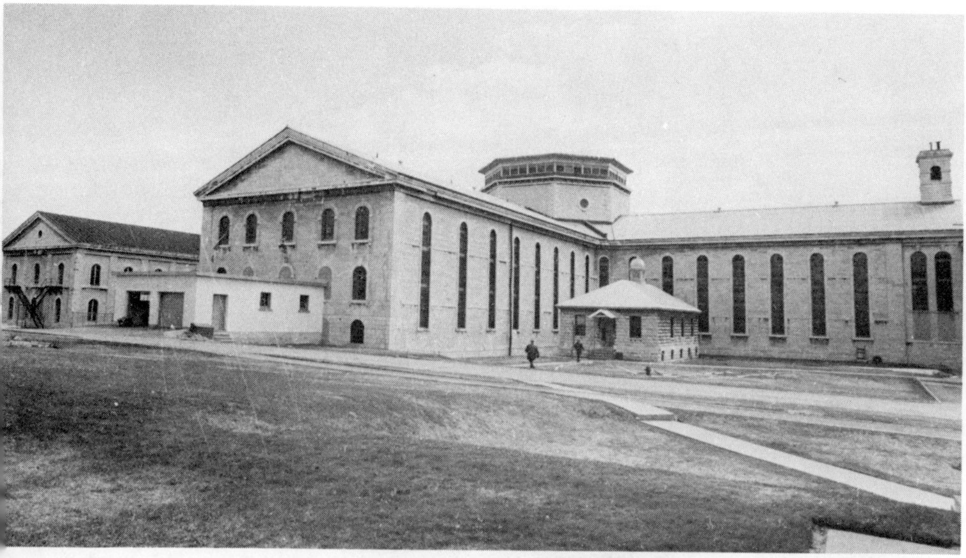

Kingston
Penitentiary – Riot
Day, April 14,
1971.
Kingston Whig-Standard)

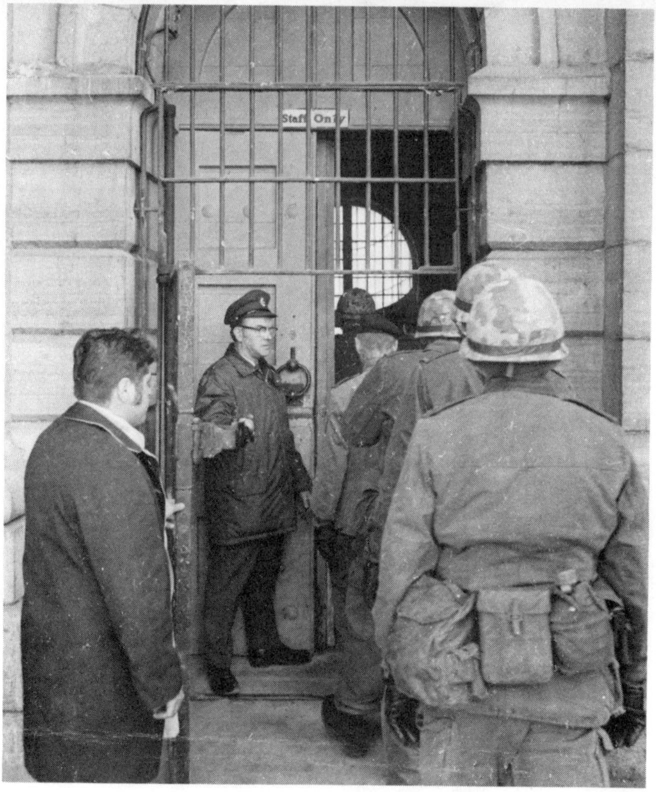


ldiers arrive at
e gate of
ingston
enitentiary to
tablish a security
rimeter around
e riot area.
ngston Whig-Standard)

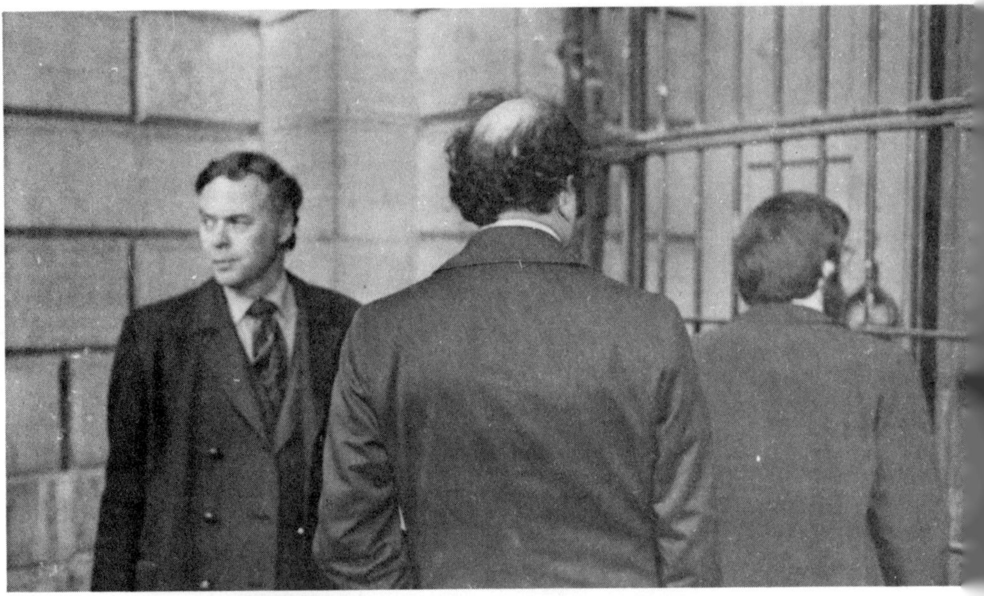

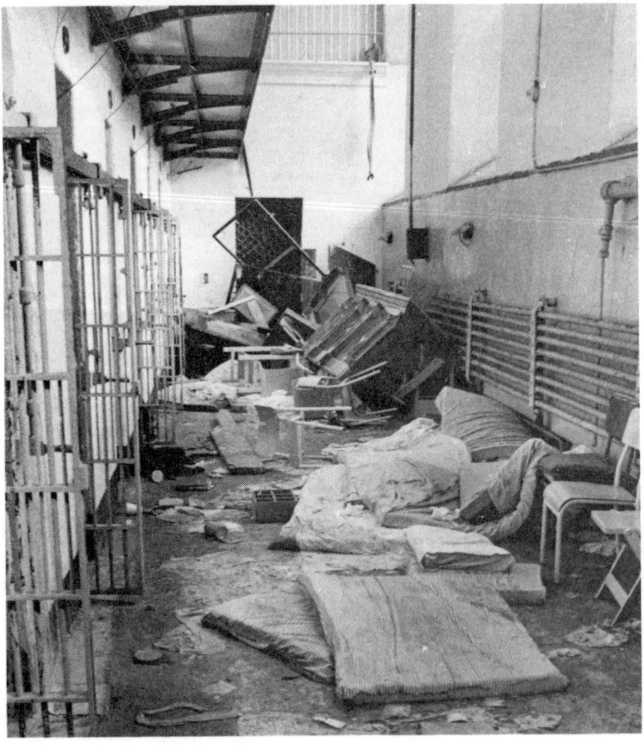

*Mediators arriving upon inmates' request.*
(Kingston Whig-Standar

*Wreckage of cell area where sexua offenders were housed.*
(Kingston Whig-Stanc

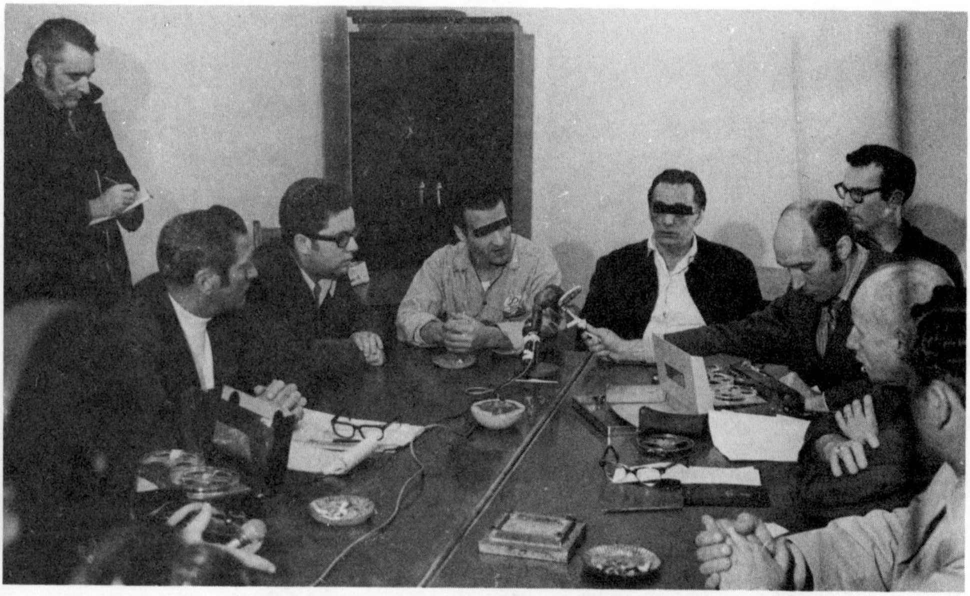

*Mediation conference between representatives of the inmate population and penitentiary officials.*
*(Kingston Whig-Standard)*

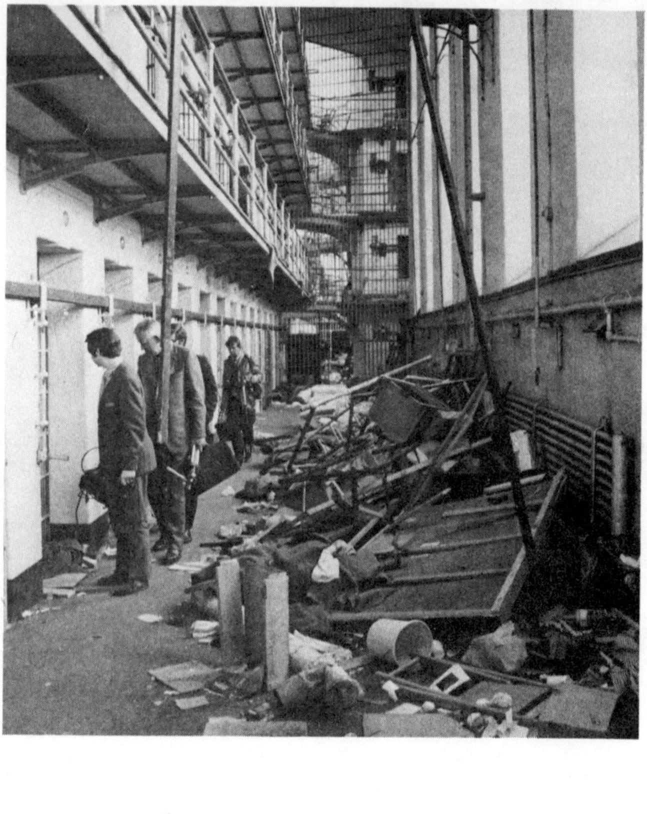

*Vreckage thrown om the four tiers cells facing the ntral area.*
*ingston Whig-Standard)*

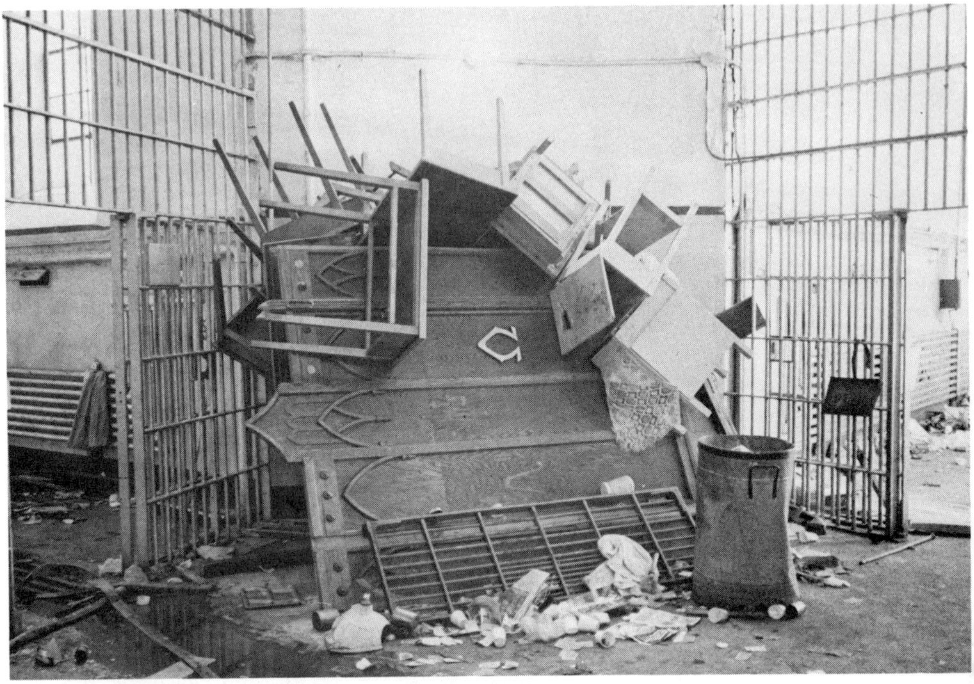

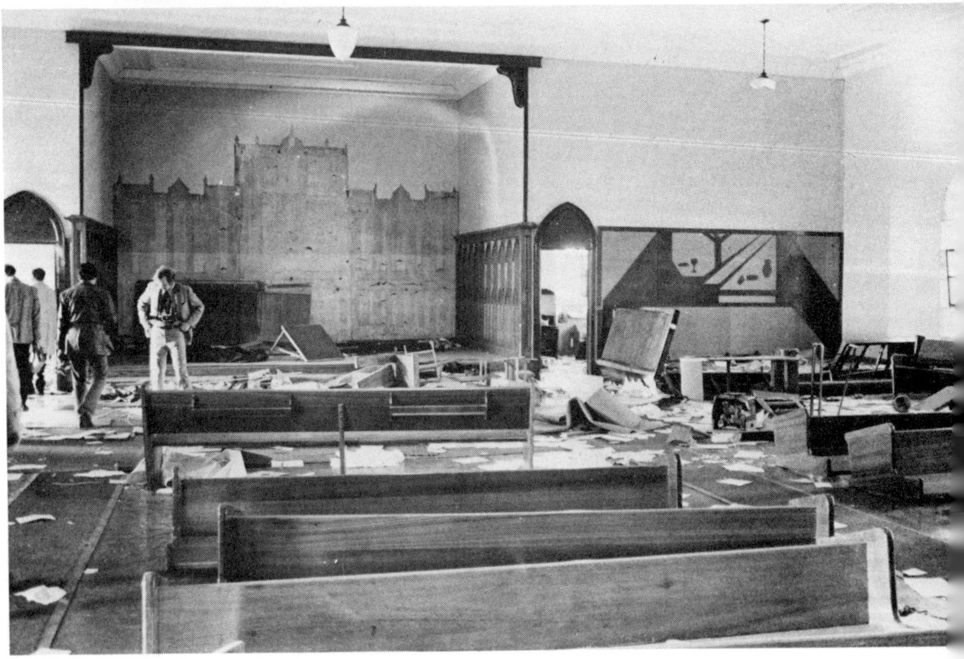

*Chapel furniture thrown off the chapel landing. (upper left)*
*(Kingston Whig-Standard)*

*Wreckage of the prison chapel. (lower left)*
*(Kingston Whig-Standard)*

*Iron bar ripped from its socket to gain access to sex offenders cells. (upper right)*
*(Kingston Whig-Standard)*

*Cell from which an unnamed inmate was dragged to his "trial". (lower right)*
*Kingston Whig-Standard)*

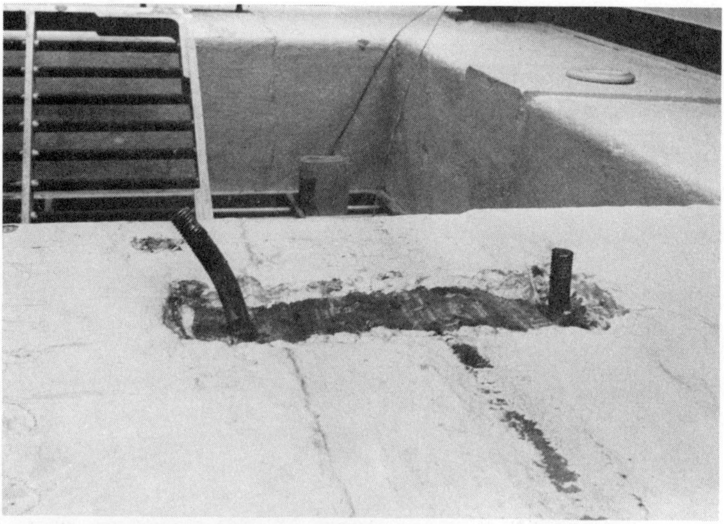

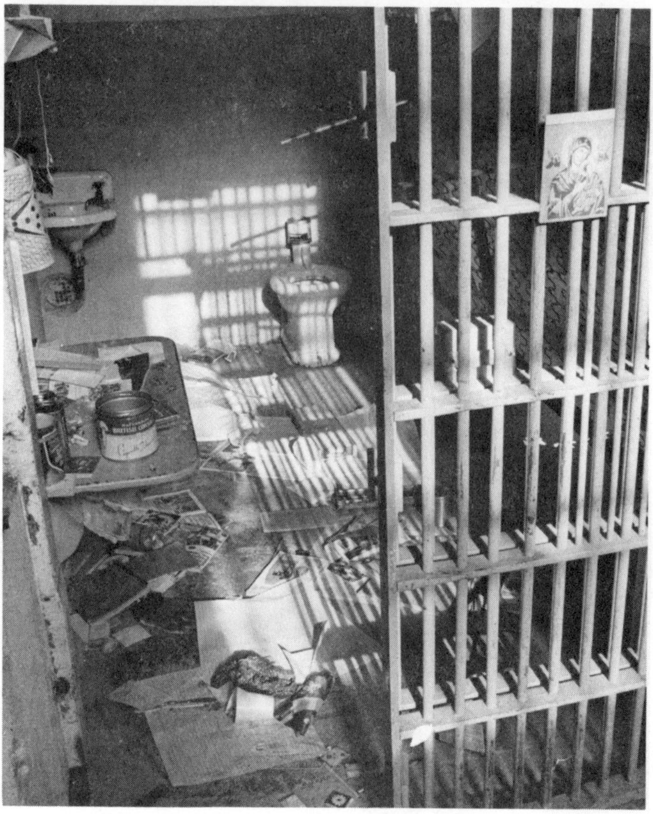

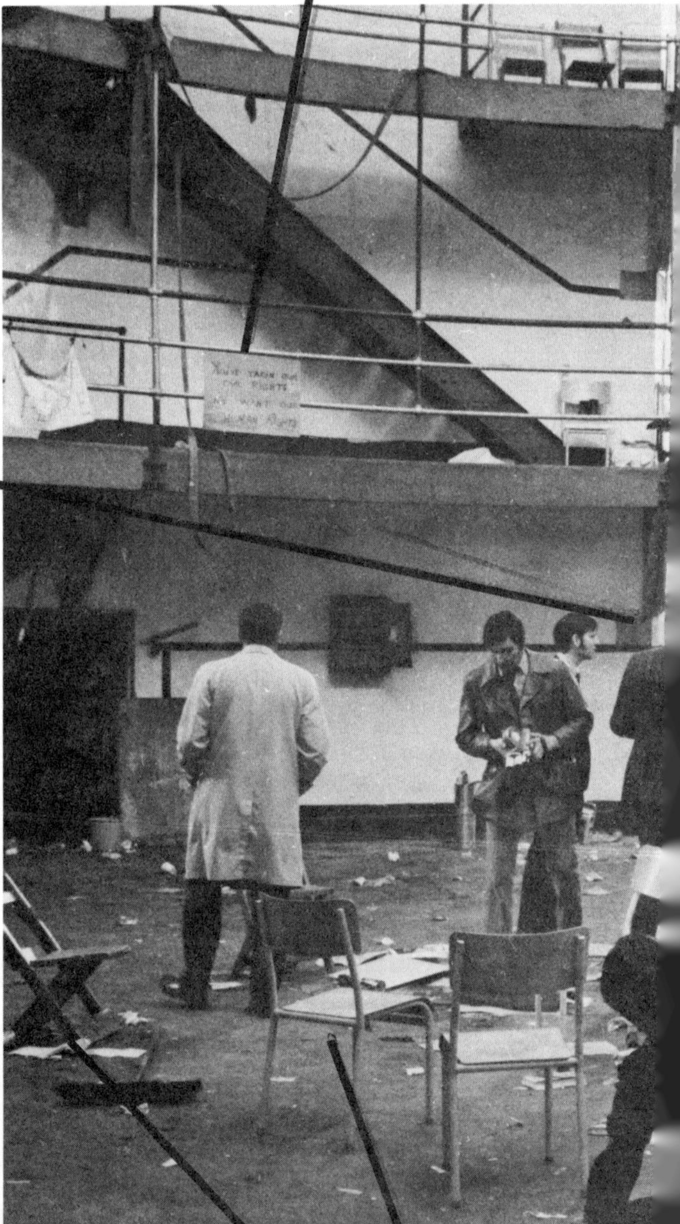


*Chairs arranged in a circle around the centre of the rotunda, where inmates were beaten in an orgy of physical destruction during the mock trial.*

*(Kingston Whig-Standard)*

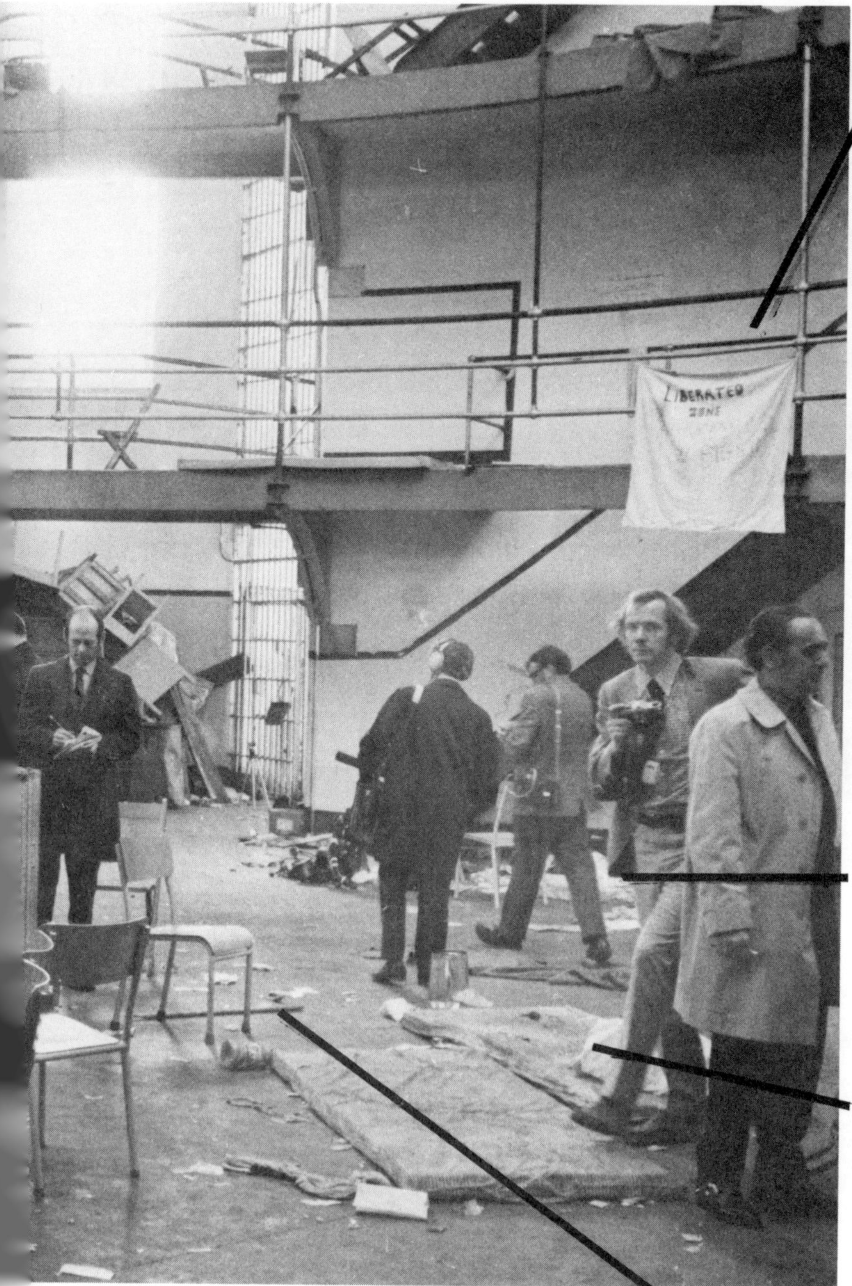


LIBERATED ZONE
FOR HUMAN PIGS

SHEETS USED
TO COVER
INMATES IN
DEATH RING

VICTIM'S SHEET
AND MATTRESS

INSTRUMENT OF DEATH
– AN IRON BAR

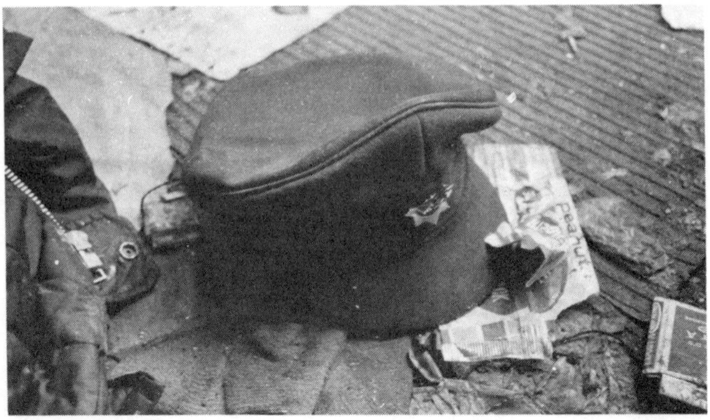

*Cap and jacket of Correctional Officer Flynn lying on the floor of the fourth tier.*
(Kingston Whig-Standard)

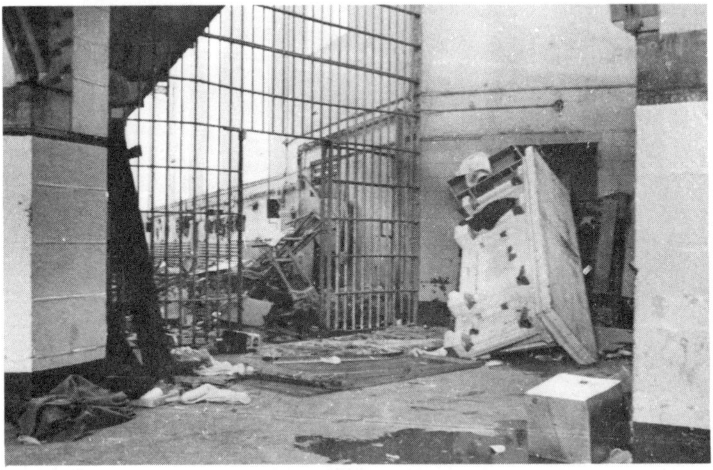

*A chesterfield from the chapel lounge.*
(Kingston Whig-Standard)

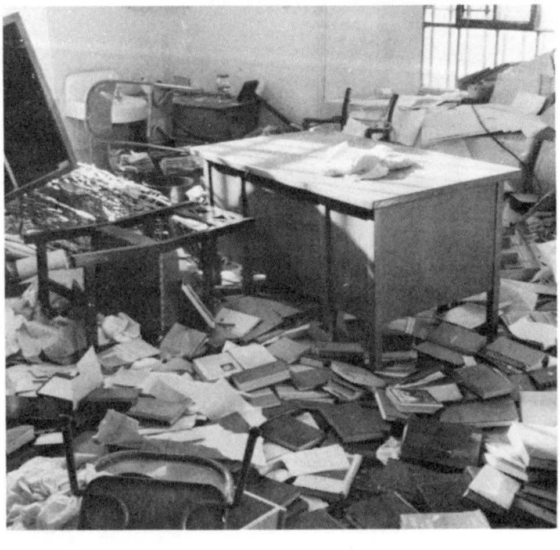

*Padre's office hewn with prayer books and other reading material.*
(Kingston Whig-Standard

this, that, and the other thing. But fundamentally, they are suspicious of the world. They don't trust people. They keep feeling something is wrong. Thinking that people are against them, they nurture a persecution complex. "The boss has got it in for me," is a familiar complaint. "Nobody treats me fairly," is another.

The schizoid, cyclothymic and paranoid personalities basically are normal reactions to the world. Every normal person has a tendency in one of these directions. Some of us are simply not influenced to any degree by changes in the world and others are profoundly affected. And some of us are suspicious of everything around us, people and events, and interpret them only in terms of ourselves.

Understanding these categories of normal people provides a basis for understanding the categories into which abnormal people may be grouped, for abnormal people tend to express mental illness in terms of what their basic personality types were before their illnesses took control of them.

The schizoid personality, with his indrawn, quiet, mind-my-own-business attitude, his engrossed-in-his-own-thoughts characteristic, and his desire to straighten things out on his own, develops, when he becomes mentally ill, into a schizophrenic. A schizophrenic's illness is typified by a withdrawal from the world around him. He will sit in a chair for hours and not communicate in any way. A great deal may be going on inside this personality but normal functioning has ceased because the mind and emotions have closed down to the outside world.

When the cyclothymic personality becomes mentally ill, he becomes a manic depressive. Manic means over-active, and depressive means under-active. Manic depressives go either all out, or all under. The manic is hyper. He becomes so over-active that he can't sit still. He is impressed with everything, is talkative and continually generating ideas, many of which are unreasonable. One man I knew startled everyone by buying two airplanes for himself. The strange part of the purchase was not particularly that he bought two planes but that he didn't know how to fly. The depressive, on the other hand, sinks into depression. He gives up easily, saying, for example, "There's no point to life." He is a potential suicide victim.

The paranoid person, when he becomes mentally ill, develops a condition called paranoia, which produces an acute feeling of persecution that often leads to violence against others. It is easy to see how such a condition can develop when the person continually believes he is being followed or that other people are prying into and influencing his affairs.

Ultimately, the mentally ill paranoid decides he has had enough persecution and actually resorts to violence. He is a dangerous person.

**The Mental Defective Personality**

A fourth type of personality is the retarded individual whose mental equipment is incomplete. His behavior is inconsistent and, to a considerable extent, unpredictable because his mind doesn't function along normal lines, even under the best of conditions.

This classification of personalities is basically simple. It is also accurate. Individuals are either ingoing or outoing, hostile, or mentally defective. All of these types are present in penal institutions, as indeed everywhere else. Schizophrenics in prison are withdrawn. They don't want anyone around and consequently are of little danger to others. Manic depressives are also quiet and withdrawn if depressed, and liable to commit suicide. Though not many manics are found behind bars, these people are usually quite pleasant. They are so busy fussing around, busying themselves with all kinds of things, that they never become involved in serious trouble. They occasionally cause damage but this is unintentional and they never hurt anyone. Paranoid people are as suspicious in prison as out of it. They don't like their custodians, and are constantly saying things like, "You're on my back," and "What have you got against me?"

This system of classification stresses the way in which an individual reacts to his surroundings, and out of it has grown the psychiatric vocabulary that describes the emotional reactions of people. It is the system that has put David in the category of "aggressive," and Wayne in that of "passive aggressive." But now let us examine the other categories.

There is also a quiet type of person who never threatens anyone, never pounds his desk, is always nice to everyone, and yet is determined that, come what may, he will get his way. I call him a manipulator because, fundamentally, this is precisely what he is. He manipulates the world around him. It's usually impossible to point your finger at him and say, "You did such-and-such a thing." Yet you know that somehow he managed to bring about the situation you are talking about. He falls into the aggressive-passive group which is not to be confused with the passive-aggressive category. The aggressive we are talking about here is quiet and subtle and can be very smooth-talking.

Prisons have had their quotas of these so-called "nice guys," the pitchmen with some pretty convincing pitches. The shady automobile salesman is almost a stereotypic example of this group. They are the people who, as criminals, are involved in fraud, false pretenses and misrepresentation. They are the sharpies, the confidence men. They don't stick up banks and run the risk of being shot in a police chase. That is too dangerous. They would rather con the manager with a cheque than hold up a teller with a gun.

I am thinking of one old con artist who was very smooth in his younger days. He'd walk into a bank and immediately ask to see the manager. Well-dressed and highly personable, he would tell the manager that he was passing through town when his car broke down. He had a cheque from a company for which he said he worked, and would appreciate it if he could cash it. Well, the banker should have been more cautious but he wasn't. Glancing at the man's credentials (he had all kinds of identification, most of it printed for him by a friend), the manager would scribble his initials on the cheque and the man would pick up his money from a teller. The cheque, of course, would bounce shortly thereafter. This was a highly successful holdup but the thief, being an aggressive-passive, would hold up the bank in a subtle, non-violent way.

Then there is Murray, who has managed to stay on the street only four of the last thirteen years. It seems to me a smart con man would have a better batting average but it doesn't seem to bother him. He has been in my office at K.P. numerous times, for evaluations, problem discussions and what-have-you and, each time, I get the feeling that here's a man who really enjoys his work, risks notwithstanding.

"I get along well with people, that's the secret," he confided one day. "For some reason or other, people seem to like me. I'll go into a completely strange town and in a couple of weeks, I know everybody and everybody knows me. And here's the thing, they all think I'm a hell of a nice guy. It's play-acting, really. You know, you pretend you're a college boy looking for work, or you're a young fellow who's just lost his wife. You work out a scenario and you stick with it."

Murray went into an Ontario town on one occasion as head of a fictitious company called Home Discount Imports, which supposedly imported Japanese radios and certain electronic equipment, and walked away a month later with seven thousand dollars. He was flat broke to start with and didn't even have a sample radio as a come-on. But he and a woman who posed as his wife moved into a brand new apartment house, rented an office downtown and ordered several hundred dollars worth of ping pong tables and basketball equipment for a new YMCA branch which had just been opened. The sporting goods firm agreed to bill him later. It took three weeks to set up the town, he was proud to reveal. By then he had been accepted as a bona fide businessman – and as a philanthropist by the YMCA. Then he began asking people to cash cheques for him, and some of them did. They were worthless, of course, but before they could bounce back, he was gone.

Murray has no remorse. "I'm a cheque-passer, okay," he says, "but I have no sympathy for the people who accept them. It's their own stupidity and greed. You go into a store and you buy something and you ask them to take a cheque because you have no cash. Well, if they're going to accept a cheque from a stranger, that's their hard luck. It's greed, you see. They'll take a chance on the cheque rather than run the risk of losing a sale."

In prison, manipulators like Murray have to be watched carefully. They are usually more intelligent and better educated than other inmates and make a point of cooperating with the administration for the sake of preferential treatment and good jobs.

There is a type of person who is always thinking about his own personal satisfaction. This is what we call a dependent personality. A criminally-inclined dependent, timid in personality by nature, is likely to become involved in offences that carry with them high emotional rewards. The offences usually have to do with things they desire impulsively. Sexual offences are high on the list. Dependents are also drug addicts, alcoholics and arsonists. One of the inmates who came to see me was a man who had been propositioned by a homosexual, a barber's assistant, in civilian life. Angered and disgusted, he had returned to the barber shop later and set fire to it.

The dependent personality has no initiative and keeps looking for a recipe for good behavior. He will cause no trouble if he is with the right crowd but he will follow anyone who gives him attention. When I questioned one of these inmates about how he got along in the institution, he replied, "I mind my own business and obey the rules the best I can."

Another category includes what we call the inadequate personality. People in this group are unable to cope with their environment, on the street or behind bars. They are emotionally defective individuals, perhaps mentally retarded. Their offences are usually of a minor nature. They will be arrested for simple theft, for example. Occasionally, they will be accused of indecent assault.

"Have you learned anything in the institution?" I asked one young inmate, serving time for theft.

"Honestly sir, no," he answered. "I am very easily defeated. If somebody says something, or something happens, I get discouraged and I sort of draw into myself."

A few inmates are on what I call the edge of sanity. It is difficult to draw the line between those who should be in a penitentiary and those who should be in a mental institution. The mentals have to be watched all the time. They are picked on, and made fun of, by other inmates and some are definite suicide risks.

"I feel that people dislike me," one man confided. "If I went for a job or anything, I felt...well, they don't want no part of me, they don't want to help me. Then I'd get disgusted and do something, like stealing, forging cheques."

"Do you find that when you're alone there are...well, let's say unnatural ideas going through your head...a voice perhaps?" I asked.

"Continuously. I'm told to do things. So-and-so is against you. So-and-so is going to get you. Sometimes, I hear what's going to happen, what way they're going to get me. I'm told to do away with myself. Quite often I have it in mind because there is nothing to look forward to here in this institution. When I get out...well, I'll be back. I know that, so I have nothing to lose."

Some time later, this inmate was brought into the prison medical wing, writhing in pain. He had broken a razor blade in half and placed the two pieces in a small chunk of doughy white bread. He had then wet the bread so that it would hold together and swallowed it. When the bread finally dissolved, the pieces of razor began cutting away at his stomach lining. He was rushed to Kingston General Hospital, where surgeons operated and removed the offending metal.

It is also possible to cross-catalogue personalities, drawing a more accurate picture of an individual with mixed characteristics. An example of one such case is an inmate of Joyceville Institution who, one night a few years ago, when he was twenty-two years old, got drunk, held up a bar and frightened the hell out of the customers by firing a gun in the air several times. Though he was intoxicated at the time of the incident, the judge gave him a fourteen-year sentence. This man has the typical schizoid profile: quiet, withdrawn, reluctant to involve himself intimately with other people. You'd never think of him as a wild western-style gunman – yet, fundamentally, he is an angry and aggressive man.

Indeed, almost without exception, the crime fits the personality of the person who has committed it. When the crime pattern varies, we must look for reasons. The pattern reflects consistencies in behavior, or alterations in behavior, in much the same fashion as the psychological projection tests, the Rorschach group. The pattern also mirrors age variables in the rise and fall of aggressive statistics. We know, for instance, that the period of maximum aggression potential is between twenty and forty years of age. From forty to sixty years of age, the criminal goes into a stage of decline, with reduced aggression, and from sixty on, he is considered to be in a state of senile dependency and vegetative in nature. It has been said that there are no old men in prison. This is not entirely true. There are some. Most criminals reach a point of maturity at some time or other and decide they've had enough of crime. Maturity? Well, yes, though maturity and infirmity sometimes go hand in hand. As one inmate once remarked, "I'm getting too old for that stuff now."

The crime pattern is a useful tool for projecting future criminal activity. It is precise enough to indicate a variety of erratic behavior in the criminal makeup. Our knowledge has enabled us to place inmates in particular categories. We are able to classify people like the Davids and Waynes of our penitentiary populations. We know their characteristics, their personality conflicts.

The aggressive and passive-aggressive personalities carry their identities into the prison culture and form its core, the aggressives being the leaders, the passive-aggressives the followers. They are both adverse to all prison administration responsibilities. The aggressive-passive people will accept such responsibilities and won't usually identify with aggressive groups. Dependent inmates are rejected by the prison culture and live a fringe life. They still seek their satisfactions in emotional outlets, usually of a homosexual nature. Defectives live as simply as they can, trusted by one one and helped by no one. The mentally-disturbed, separated by their own illness processes, often develop deep resentments and become extreme problems in management and discipline.

Criminals are predictable. Holdup men don't usually play con games. The break-and-entry boys don't stick up banks. If I find a man with a record of widely-divergent offences such as, say, holdup, break-and-entry, vagrancy, car theft and sexual assault, I immediately assume he is mentally disturbed. An inconsistent crime pattern reflects a seriously-disturbed, pre-psychotic individual.

Inmates can be better handled when they are properly identified. For example, one inmate was involved in sexual offences, based on a particular delusion that he should teach ten-year-old boys how to become sexually active. He is now serving a long sentence for contributing to juvenile delinquency and knowlege of his personality orientation can help immensely in dealing with him. Basically, this man believes that he should not be in an institution. He feels the officers are persecuting him and he is continually writing letters to the authorities, attempting to gain his release.

Another inmate, who comes from the Middle East, has written a number of letters to Prime Minister Trudeau, complaining that he has been brainwashed in the prison system. When he is released, he says, he is going to blow up the Canadian Embassy – and the American Embassy as well – because he believes he has been persecuted in North America. An individual such as this must be watched carefully. An inmate with a persecution complex can make it very difficult for everybody, for his is a dangerous personality.

**CHAPTER 9**

# Murderers I Have Known

The word spreads quickly inside the walls: there's a new guy on the range. Another murderer has joined the captive community – and if this *fish* thinks he's going to slip anonymously into the shadows, he's wrong. The population knows who he is and what he's done. What's more, it passed its own judgment on him long before his actual admission.

"He knocked off a security guard."

The word filters down the grapevine. There is no need for comment. Everybody knows it's a case of something having gone wrong. You don't kill a guard for the fun of it. No more than you'd kill a shopkeeper, or a service station attendant, or a building superintendent. You're playing a dangerous game – and those are the breaks. Tough shit.

"He's a cop killer."

This man isn't going to hit it off too well inside. He will have no status whatever in the institution. Every inmate knows that when you kill a cop, you get the bulls mad, and when the bulls get mad the heat's on all over town. They'll nab every guy they can lay their hands on – even if it's only for spitting on the sidewalk. No, you never shoot a policeman. Never.

"He blew away his old lady."

Judgment will be reserved in this case. As it would be with the Prison for Women inmate who blew away her old man. There are always two sides to domestic quarrels. Nagging wives, drunken husbands. Who knows where it all started. When you don't know the people involved, or the problems, just stay well out of it because you don't know what you're talking about. And that's the truth.

"The creep strangled a kid."

This individual is in trouble right from Day One. Five packs of cigarettes says somebody's going to go looking for him before long. If the authorities haven't put him in segregation already, he'd better ask for a reservation there immediately.

"He's a nut and shouldn't be here."

This man hasn't been declared insane but everybody in the joint knows he isn't playing with a full deck. Most inmates feel sorry for him but then what can you do for a guy who's lost some of his marbles? Nothing. Just leave him alone. Let him do his own time.

Murderers account for about ten per cent of the Canadian penitentiary population at any given time. At this writing, there are some nine hundred behind bars, serving life sentences for first and second degree murder. Another four hundred are incarcerated after conviction on the lesser offence of manslaughter.

Murder is in the first degree when it is planned and deliberate, when the victim is a policeman or prison employee, and when it is committed during a hijacking, kidnapping, or act of rape or indecent assault on a female. Under the life sentence imposed here, the offender may not apply for parole until he has served a minimum of twenty-five years.

Murder in the second degree, in broad, general terms, is one that was not planned or deliberate. The life sentence here requires that an offender serve at least ten years before applying for parole, though a sentencing judge may extend the period by a number of years.

Manslaughter is defined by the Criminal Code as a culpable homicide that would have been murder if the person who committed it had not acted in the "heat of passion caused by sudden provocation." The fact of drunkenness may also be a consideration in reducing a charge of murder to one of manslaughter. A person so convicted is liable to imprisonment for life but actual time served may be as little as five years.

Convicted murderers move into the prison system in much the same way as other people found guilty of criminal acts. They are accepted and integrated into the prison culture, or rejected by it, in accordance with the judgment of their fellow inmates.

Murderers are not special people in an institution. No special than they were on the outside.

I tend to think of murderers as "ordinary" people. This, of course, is a wide (and highly debatable) generalization. After all, some of them hold up banks, others are muggers and a few are rapists.

My studies over the years, however, indicate tht half of all murders and manslaughters are family-related. The relation may be immediate, as in the case of a wife or husband-killing; or more remote, as in cases involving cousins and nephews.

They are ordinary people. And these ordinary people commit half the country's homicides.

Books and movies have given us an image of murderers as people of great cunning and expertise who plan their dastardly crimes with meticulous attention to detail and whose scenarios are as exotic as they are inventive. The cool killer of popular detective fiction does exist, of course, and some true-life murders have been as imaginative as any our good writers have been able to come up with. But these cases are really not common.

Most murderers are people who have been caught up in circumstances which had led them into murder and only an occasional inmate states, "If I were in the same situation again, I'd do the same thing."

Murder is a stone's throw away from any one of us at any time, as assailant or victim.

Murder can happen so quickly. So easily. A thin knife, a sharp letter-opener, a hatpin directed with little force in the area of the heart and life can come to an end. Suddenly.

I remember the words of one inmate I saw. He said, "It was like cutting into six inches of butter at room temperature."

Murder is a stupid thing. I have heard this from people who have killed. But murder is not the act of a stupid person necessarily. In fact, in a group of fifty-four inmates convicted for first and second degree murder, whom I followed between 1970 and 1975, fifty per cent were of average intelligence, and thirty per cent were above average. Only twenty per cent of that group were below average.

My studies of that group produced some other interesting data. For example, alchohol was a contributing factor in sixty per cent of the homicides. It is worth noting, too, that only thirty per cent had previous criminal records, a statistic that supports my claim that most murders are committed by ordinary people. My inmates reported poor childhood situations, forty-eight per cent of them coming from broken homes, and fourteen per cent of them from hostile homes.

Twenty per cent of the group had previous history of mental illness. Interestingly enough, however, only a small percentage required psychiatric assistance while in prison. The old saying that time heals all wounds holds true as much inside the walls as outside. I have seen inmates in states of extreme remorse, individuals who believed their lives had been shattered beyond repair because of their actions. But man was not intended to suffer remorse forever. It's a psychological fact that it takes two to three years to get over a normal bereavement in free society. It takes a convicted murderer about the same time to get over his remorse.

**CHAPTER 10**

# Murder in the Early, Middle and Later Years

Homicide is spelled out clearly in the Canadian Criminal Code:

"A person commits homicide when, directly or indirectly, by any means, he causes the death of a human being.

Homicide is culpable or not culpable.

Homicide that is not culpable is not an offence.

Culpable homicide is murder or manslaughter or infanticide.

A person commits culpable homicide when he causes the death of a human being:

(a) by means of an unlawful act,

(b) by criminal negligence,

(c) by causing that human being, by threats or fear of violence, or by deception, to do anything that causes his death, or

(d) by wilfully frightening that human being, in the case of a child or sick person."

The law is specific. It sees the physical crime and prescribes the punishment that fits. We psychiatrists aren't satisfied to stop there. We want to know why someone is murdered. Of course, we are operating from the premise that people are primarily instinctual, that they are basically emotional creatures. They can act logically, or illogically, but logic is a variable commodity since it can be fashioned to satisfy the emotional quality of the individual.

Murder is a psychological affair. Normal psychological impulses can be converted by circumstance into abnormal mental reactions and suddenly the stage is set for murder. An unhappy combination of circumstances, coupled with a certain set of emotional and mental characteristics on the part of an individual can produce fatal results, as will be demonstrated in the cases chosen for this chapter.

Criminologists have classified murder in a great many ways over the years but I will deal with it in terms of age groups. There are certain patterns to murder and they vary greatly with maturity. When an eighteen-year-old commits murder, his motivation likely will be different from that of a thirty, or forty, or fifty-year-old. Let us think then of murder in the three great cycles of life: the early years, the middle years and the after years.

* * *

**Murder in the early years**

Robbery sets the scene for many murders among people in their teens and twenties. A shopkeeper resists, for example, and is shot. A good Samaritan citizen goes to the aid of someone who is being robbed and receives a fatal bullet wound. A taxi driver screams out for help and his fare in the back seat caves in his skull.

Our society is attuned to sudden death. It's what psychiatrists call being "death aware." Sudden death in all its dimensions is the daily diet of newspapers. It is sensational news in all communities, big or small. It is an event which stirs the curiosity of people, even fascinating them at times. We have come to accept murder which is incidental to robbery. We are alarmed, however, by senseless violence.

Murderers under the age of twenty can be very vicious during the act of robbing someone. A victim who chides them about their threats, who makes disparaging remarks, who touches, accidentally or otherwise, a raw nerve may stir up some great pent-up rage in the aggressors and precipitate wildly bizarre action.

Take the case of Billy, an eighteen-year-old with an unusual capacity for hate.

Billy, hitchkiking on Highway 2 in southern Ontario in May of 1972, was picked up by a thirty-five-year-old commercial artist who was a homosexual. During the course of the drive, the man showed him photographs of young men performing sexual acts. Later, turning off onto a side road and coming to a stop in a secluded area, he propositioned him.

When the man touched him, Billy reached for an empty pop bottle on the floor and hit him over the head with it. He pulled the dazed man out of the car and tied his hands together with rope he found in the luggage compartment. He then tied him by the wrists to the back bumper of the vehicle and dragged him over the gravel side roads until the arms were dismembered from the body.

Billy left the remains under a culvert, drove the victim's car to a nearby hotel and spent the afternoon in the bar. Police found the body later and began investigating. It was not long before they checked on the car Billy had left standing in the hotel parking lot. Bartenders recalled that a new patron had been drinking there on the day of the murder and described him. Three days later, police arrested him, questioned him and charged him with murder.

His arrest and subsequent trial were big events in the community and public opinion went strongly in favor of Billy. One individual went so far as to refer to him in a newspaper interview as "that poor Christian boy," an innocent who had been molested by a homosexual. Actually, that "poor Christian boy" was not poor. He came from an average, fairly well-to-do middle-class family.

Billy had two older sisters who bossed him around, continually placing him in the little brother role. He developed a quiet, withdrawn personality and resorted to daydreaming. At school, he made only passing marks and his teacher described him as a quiet, sad person. Billy himself admitted that he had daydreamed in angry thoughts since the age of ten.

He had fantasies and they were of revenge killings, torturing his sisters and harming his teachers. His mood was cold and factual. He didn't enjoy contact with people because he was preoccupied with the thought drama in his head of fighting back at those who belittled him. He was convicted of murder in the second degree and arrived at Kingston Penitentiary a hostile, self-contained, isolated and angry youth.

These youthful offenders are identified by the bizarre nature of their offences, their cold-eyed contempt for everyone and their preoccupation with violent fantasy. The murderous act is triggered by some situation which threatens the precarious balance of their self-esteem. With Billy, who had trained himself to exist and function without emotion, the thought of a person considering him to be homosexual was more than he was able to bear. That thought was the trigger point of what was a remorseless murder.

In a catastrophic fifteen seconds, the aggression, loosened through his feeling of panic and terror over his sexual identity, destroyed a human life.

Billy's behavior was not altered by prison, as his street personality fitted easily into the society of inmates. After some five years, he matured and his personality became more confident and assertive. He was placed in a position of respect by his fellow inmates, became a force on the inmate committee, and in 1974 led a sit-down strike. In 1975, he was judged ready for day parole and full parole followed soon after. He is currently working as a truck driver in the Toronto area and all indications are that he is living up to his responsibilities as a good, law-abiding, contributing citizen.

Diagnostically, Billy was not mentally ill, although his emotions had been bitter with rage since childhood. His mental functions certainly were very close to those of the mentally disturbed schizophrenic but for the sake of diagnosis, I call these cold, young men with their penchant for bizarre crime, pre-psychotic schizophrenics.

Murder is always an act of the mind. In Billy's case, his mental content became fixed in an angry, unrelenting drama of hate towards the world. People in this group have clear-cut psychological fears, frustrations and conflicts which may lead to murder under certain aggravations. Billy's whole image was threatened, suddenly and unexpectedly, when the driver of the car suggested a homosexual act. When he reached for the pop bottle, it was with colossal rage. No one must think of him as homosexual. No one.

* * *

Murderers, in their earlier years, all have strong mental components of hostility and fantasy. All are quiet, isolated people who have no warm contact with anyone. They live within themselves until, at some moment in time, their minds are turned inside-out, so to speak, to produce impulsive, uncontrolled acts devoid of feeling or sentiment.

No one can be sure when such a trigger action will take place but friends and acquaintances will remark with conviction afterward, "I knew it would happen sometime." The story of Craig and Jimmy are in my files under "role playing." In 1961, they staged a real-life game and, for the sake of realism, killed their principal player.

Craig and Jimmy were both seventeen and in the twelfth grade in high school. They were raised in middle class homes by parents who were kindly and supportive. They themselves, however, maintained a subtle estrangement from their parents and did not confide their feelings. The boys were known to everyone in their southern Ontario home town as quiet, well-behaved teenagers. Their schooling was satisfactory but they had no interest in sports. Their teachers noted that they were inseparable friends who shared their company with no one. They skied together, hunted rabbits together and spent long periods every evening talking to each other on the telephone. Like all normal boys, they enjoyed hobbies. Craig liked music and played the drums. Jimmy was an avid reader and enjoyed murder stories. You would have had to say that, by and large, they were a couple of pretty nice, well-adjusted kids.

Thus Craig's and Jimmy's parents received the shock of their lives when Ontario Provincial Police advised them they were charging the boys with murder.

On the evening of Remembrance Day, November 11, a police patrol car pulled over to the shoulder on a lonely stretch of Highway 401 to check out a stationary car. Training their flashlights on the interior of the vehicle, officers made a grisly discovery. The body of an adult male was slumped over the steering wheel with five bullet holes in the back of his head, each neatly an inch apart.

There had been some light snow that day and police picked up the trail of fresh footprints. They followed them across a field to another highway, where they found two boys trying to hitch a ride. They spoke to them and, instinctively suspicious, detained them for questioning. By early morning, they were preparing murder charges against Craig and Jimmy in the killing of a twenty-six-year-old man neither of them knew.

I was called into the case when one of Canada's famed criminal lawyers asked me to assess Jimmy's mental status. My examination involved three separate interviews in the local jail, with Jimmy agreeing to a "narco analysis," a psychiatric technique that reduces conscious control in a patient and makes it possible to determine the truth of certain statements.

Jimmy cooperated fully. He said that he and Craig had planned the whole thing. They would hitch a ride in a car whose only occupant was the driver, shoot the motorist, steal his money and make off with his car. The first car that stopped was a Volkswagen and the affable driver said, "Hop in, boys." Craig, Jimmy said, got into the back seat and pulled out his gun and it was pop, pop, pop, pop, pop. Five little bullets, all in a row. In detail, in three separate sessions, he related the identical story of the shooting.

Craig refused to become involved with psychiatry. He decided he'd tell his story to his lawyer instead. It was the same story Jimmy had told me – in every detail but one. When the Volks pulled to a stop, it was Jimmy who got into the back seat. And Jimmy who pressed the trigger.

The statements raised a problem in trial procedure. Would the Crown charge each one separately, which is the usual practice, or charge one as the principal and the other as an accomplice? Since both denied their guilt, and each accused the other, it appeared the boys had produced a clever stalemate.

The Crown finally decided to charge them jointly with murder. In the course of the trial, evidence was introduced that the boys had planned a railroad station robbery as well. Police even uncovered rough drawings of the layout of a station with notes on train arrival times and the movement of mail to downtown banks and offices. Both maintained the robbery plans weren't serious. It was just a "pretend idea," Craig said, to give them something to talk about.

The jury found them guilty of first degree murder but, because of their youth, the court handed down a life sentence for each, with parole eligibility in about ten years. And on March 28, 1962, Craig and Jimmy, just turned eighteen, their hands in cuffs, their feet in chains, walked through the great gray doors of Kingston Penitentiary into the cold, glamourless world of losers. The games were over. The curtain was down. Each now had to learn to survive with his nature skills, his wits – and always the fearful thought that, without help from anyone, he might not survive the curse of captivity.

In prison, they lost their closeness for one another. As time went on, they refused even to talk about one another, except to reiterate that the other was guilty. Jimmy learned to accept prison routine and cooperated with custodial staff, and after twenty-two months was considered suitable for a medium security institution. His friend pursued another course. He was irritable, offered only passive cooperation and sometimes made veiled threats about Jimmy. Psychiatrically, there was no evidence of mental disease, both personalities being stable and consistent within their own patterns. Over the years, however, Craig became more defensive and distant, while Jimmy practiced an ongoing attitude of cooperation toward both staff and shop work.

Craig and Jimmy were finally paroled and now, twenty years after the crime, are leading apparently normal lives. Craig with his cool, organized, expressive personality is gainfully employed in the large earth-moving machine business. Jimmy is a bookkeeper. Married, with two children, he is now a productive member of a small community.

Insanity? No. The crime was a bizarre extension of the "pretend period" of childhood. Many children, left to themselves, with no playmates, find amazing friends in the rain pipe, the cupboard, the cellar. Daydreaming, imagining, fantasy and preoccupation provide psychological relief from the boredom of many a child's day.

Role playing is obvious in the cops and robbers game, the cowboys and Indians of other years. Identification with the good guy or the bad guy becomes stronger if the person is, within himself, lonely, bored and unhappy. He says to himself: a colorful personality is added to my life if, for a period of time, I become someone else.

In this particular case, the two boys developed an emotional hunger for adventure. Both had cautious and limited relationships with their families. Both were uninterested in sports. They were inclined to be loners and complemented one another in reinforcing their loneliness and isolation from other people.

As their childhood and boyhood friendship developed, they shared, through dreams, not hopes of a profession or trade but thoughts of adventure as, perhaps, Billy the Kid or John Dillinger might have done. In retrospect, I can see a kind of Bonnie and Clyde drama in the story of the boys. If one of them had been a girl, the similarity would have been marked. They planned every detail of their crime. They planned that each would say the other did the killing. They thought they would never go to jail because it would be impossible to prove who was the murderer. And after the murder, they planned to stage a robbery at the railway depot.

Role playing is a consuming identification which absolves the person from any real appreciation of the nature and consequence of his acts during the masquerade of this adopted hero.

I did a lot of personal conjecturing at the time of the crime. My favorite scenario at one point involved a person unknown, a third hitchhiker who might have been in the car too, and who might have done the shooting. What would have been the verdict had the boys laid the blame on someone unknown to them who had vanished immediately after the crime?

I use written questionnaires in cases like this and ask who, when, where, and why? But in the one I prepared for young Craig, I asked something else, "Was there another person in the car besides you two and the driver?" He answered all the questions – except that one.

Was the omission significant? I'm not prepared to say it was. Yet, coming so soon after the little scenario I developed, it seemed strange. If there had been an unidentified assailant, why would the boys not have said so? Were they threatened with murder themselves if they ever disclosed the presence of the other person? Did they decide then that they would accuse each other?

I have thought of the case many times over the years and my reasoned conclusion is that the murderer is either Craig, or Jimmy, and not a third party. Craig had made it sound so plausible that Jimmy had pulled the trigger – and Jimmy had made it sound so plausible that Craig had pulled it. It had to have been one of them. Still, unanswered questions nag away at me. Why did Craig not fill in that one empty space on the questionnaire?

* * *

Murder of a vicious and senseless nature may develop out of fantasy preoccupation with alarmingly vivid brutality. Certainly sound ideas can come from the minds of outwardly sound individuals.

The mental abnormality usually is discovered when the violent, rampaging ideas are exploded into action by some trivial remark or insult, when senseless murder without motive takes place. Cases of murder by fantasy pass through the courts from time to time at the homicide level but because there is no technical evidence of insanity, the individual's actions are looked upon as purposeful and planned. Ironically, the fantasy murderer is so obsessed with his own thoughts, that he functions in a kind of "thought capsule" rather than in a rational relationship with his surroundings.

Pierre had a home background of rejection and inadequacy and a father who beat him regularly and severely. His hate mechanism began to take form at age five when he started thinking that some day he would be strong enough to beat the hell out of his father. As he grew older, he functioned in a quiet, aloof, suspicious manner. Aggression was not obvious but his work record as a lathe operator showed him to be a poor worker. Actually, his mind was seldom on his job. It was too busy attacking father images in fantasy. For example, he was always polite to his boss but then, in the evenings at home, he would spend hours devising diabolical schemes for doing away with him. He was able to develop a hateful atmosphere in any relationship, yet no one could see his destructive potential.

Pierre was twenty-one when he exploded.

It happened in a convenience store he was robbing in Toronto. The robbery itself was insignificant. The horror of it was that Pierre killed the proprietor and then cut his tongue out with a knife. In fact, he came out of the store with it in his hand.

In Kingston Penitentiary, he directed his fantasy of hate toward the authorities. As time went on, however, he began to discuss his adolescent fantasy. He couldn't explain his crime but he remembered that the five days leading up to it were filled with job problems and personal frustrations, among them repeated hassles with his aging father who kept treating him like a child. Giving up his fantasy wasn't easy because, up until then, it was all he had. But gradually, he began to realize that he was full of destructive hate.

After three years, his anger subsided and he was sent to Penetang Institution's Mental Health Centre for complete psychiatric care. There he learned that his behavior had been the result of early life experiences.

Hate is never defined as a disease, but it is a disease and a deadly one. It can be a component of many personalities. I have seen it in the children of unloving parents. They may be adequately fed and clothed, but they are treated as objects and shown no emotional support. Even as young as seven years, some of them lack spontaneous affection, avoid people who are attentive to them and feel threatened by the slightest show of warmth and approval.

They grow into adolescence, devoid of close relationships with people. Their emotions have known only fear and eventually they develop a protective and generalized hate of everyone. To this emotional pathology is added the strength of fantasy, and hate is directed to particular people and situations. Ruminations and destructive dramas take precedence over other thoughts. They develop one true emotion, coldness. They generally are able to control their hate, so as not appear outwardly hateful to others, but inside there is a sea of simmering violence.

Pierre had been plagued with fear, loneliness, anger, a kind of emotional flatness and violent fantasy–until the day of his bizarre, destructive homocide. That was fifteen years ago: a lifetime ago, really. Prison and psychiatric hospital care helped turn him around. Today, he is in free society and maintaining a comfortable relationship with the world around him.

**Murder in the middle years**

The middle years vary according to definition. For present purposes, I shall consider them as being between thirty and fifty, that period of wage-earning, reputation-building and competitive strain. These are the years of the battles for survival – in the home, on the street, at work, and, all too often, in the courts.

Murder is not an unusual phenomenon in this age category. Often, it is related to acquisitiveness. A bank robber, for instance, kills a guard who tries to block his exit. Another kills the manager of a tobacco shop when he reaches for a telephone. These are incidental murders, incidental to the business of stealing in order to obtain the so-called necessities of life.

Murder is often related to something much more personal – possessiveness. This is mined territory. The unexploded shells lie buried just below the surface, ready to blow anytime. The groundwork for murder is laid whenever someone threatens the possessive relationship one person has for another. Add drugs or alcohol, or both, and the process may be accelerated.

Maureen knows something about this. She is doing a ten-year stretch in the Prison for Women for killing her husband. She is thirty-two and a woman of tidy figure who appears youthful in the regulation slacks and shirt. The women on her range call her "The Red Whistler" because she has red hair and because she is always whistling. Her favorite song is "The Yellow Rose of Texas" and sometimes she whistles that tune all day long. Whistling is good for her. It generates confidence.

Maureen had asked to see the psychiatrist and on her referral form she had written five words: "I want to know why." When we met, she was hoping for an answer. How could she have done this terrible thing? How could she have committed murder?

Sudden death is always tragic but it is not a personal concern to anyone until it reaches into the family circle to bring strain, sadness, blame, resentment and rage. Maureen was trying to cope with the knowledge that she had brought death into her household – and that she had brought two children into the world to share her tragedy.

Maureen was the older of two girls, a healthy youngster raised in a little village near Thessalon. She was bright, spoke both French and English and reached the twelfth grade at seventeen years of age. Her only problem really was her red hair. She had a pretty face but the orange-red tint made her stand out in any group and this embarrassed her. After leaving school, she worked as a housekeeper for two years, met a carpenter named Peter, married him and moved to northern Ontario. Over the following four years, she gave birth to two baby girls.

Maureen remembers the first four years of marriage as being happy ones. Then, at a New Year's Eve party on December 31, 1976, she sensed that her husband was unusually attentive to a neighbor named Carmen. There were frequent arguments during the next few weeks and one night Peter threw his shotgun at her and said, "If you think I'm such a bastard, shoot me, you red-headed devil. Go ahead, shoot me." Maureen decided to spend some weeks with her parents after this, but when she kept hearing reports about Peter and Carmen, she came back home. The arguments resumed with wild accusations and counter-accusations. Carmen was the centre of every quarrel.

Maureen's last two years with her husband had been punctuated with numerous beatings, tauntings and degradations. Then on the evening of March 2, 1977, frightened and frustrated by a major quarrel, she locked herself in her room with her two daughters. Peter, quite drunk, tried to break down the door and finally succeeded in smashing the lock with the butt of his shotgun. He swung into the room just as the two children went into the clothes closet to hide. Once again, he gave his terrified wife the gun. "Use it, you red-haired bitch," he shouted. "And don't forget to pull the trigger. Blow my guts out, so I have as few as you."

He raised his right hand in a firm fist to strike her. A sudden explosion shook the room. The smell of smoke, blood and flesh saturated everything. Peter lay dismembered on the floor. His wife had discharged both barrels of the gun into him, literally separating his chest from his pelvis.

Why had this terrible thing happened? How could it have happened?

She was not the kind of person to fire a gun at anyone. And yet, she had. On that fateful night, some fearful force in her triggered her finger and blew her husband into eternity. Her ongoing sensitivity about her hair may very well have been a factor. When Peter called her a "red-haired bitch," it may have been too much for her.

After three years, Maureen still hasn't been able to accept her husband's death, but she has come to realize that at the time of the murder, she feared for her safety and the safety of the children. She grieves over him but never mentions the name of Carmen.

Maureen was perky the last time I visited her. She had just received a letter from home and it was full of family news, which she enjoys more than anything else. The girls are doing well at school. One is in the fifth grade, the other in the eighth. They are living with her parents who have been very supportive all along. But the past is still part of her present. She blames herself for not having sought professional help before her problems erupted into murder. But she is focussing too, on the future. She knows that someday she will be released from prison and when that day comes, she will be expected to pick up the reins of responsibility with her children.

Life in prison isn't exactly what you'd call ideal, of course, but Maureen is making out. Some days are better than others. That's just natural. And on those days when things aren't going as well as they should, well... she just whistles an extra little tune.

* * *

Marriage is the most acceptable social arrangement, ensuring security, consistency, predictability and a coordinated milieu in which to raise the offspring of the union. But nobody ever said it necessarily has to be a happy affair.

William had a marriage full of anxiety, tension, frustration and misunderstanding and on May 8, 1973, he committed what I call an "instant" murder, one which occurs entirely without planning and which is so explosive that the assailant has no recollection of it. William was forty-nine when he bludgeoned his wife, Anna, to death.

He was dumbfounded when he consulted me the first time. "I sat at my trial for three days," he said. "The prosecution proved to the jury and to me that I had murdered my wife. I don't remember anything about it, yet I know I did it. They proved everything...why don't I know all this?" He shook his head in disbelief. "I was in jail three months before my trial and had plenty of time to remember it – but I can't."

His situation was clear to me. I had no doubts about it. He had completely repressed the memory of the death because his mind could not accept the fact that he had killed his wife.

"I hear you psychiatrists can bring back my memory." He hesitated. "Can, you, Doc? It frightens me."

"Don't you think you've suffered enough?" I asked. "You've heard it all in court. Why put yourself through a meat grinder? You can't hate yourself – and survive. I think your memory had better stay locked away in your mind."

During the next four interviews, William told me a lot about himself. The rest of the story was culled from the investigation.

William came to Canada in 1946 from Surrey, England, with his new bride, Anna. It was a honeymoon emigration. They settled in a small town in southern Ontario where William, a dye-maker, had been promised work through the recommendation of the plant for which he had worked in England. Thanks to his industry, and Anna's conservative tastes, they managed to buy a three-bedroom house on the outskirts of town. Two girls, Kimberley and Elizabeth, were born to them. William later became a shop supervisor, giving him more money and more prestige. Outwardly, this was a happy, successful family.

The girls were in their early adolescence when they first sensed strains in the family fabric.

"Mom, Dad's okay, try not to criticize him," Kimberley said one day when her mother was irritated. "He's not one to take a joke, nor to handle criticism." On another occasion, Kimberley said she worried because her father couldn't seem to get interested in anything in the evenings. "He just sits there, reads the papers, goes for a walk and then goes to bed," she told her mother. "Can't you and Daddy take a holiday together?"

The relationship between the parents grew more distant as time went on. For one thing, they didn't sleep in the same room anymore. William became impatient when asked to help with household chores. Both became silent with each other – silent but polite. There were no quarrels, no unkind comments. Their relationship was frozen. There appeared to be no feeling. When Anna started talking about making a visit home to see her aged mother, the girls were excited. They thought they could see animation and interest stirring in their parents' eyes.

Then one day, William arrived home at noon, fatigued. He had lunch, and stretched out on his bed. Shortly after one, Anna called out, "You'll have to get up, William. You've got to put the curtain rods up in the girls' room and I want to get it done before four."

William got up wearily and went into the girls' room in his stocking feet. The stepladder was already in position with the screwdriver, pliers and hammer on the bed. After two attempts to hang the rod properly, he came down the ladder with the hammer in his right hand.

"I could do better than that myself," Anna snapped angrily. "You men are all..."

Those were Anna's last words on earth. The hammer descended on her skull and buried itself deeply in the soft matter of the brain tissue.

William dragged her body to the basement and with a saw, hatchet and carving knife, cut it into twenty-eight pieces, which he put in supermarket bags. He used a garden hose to wash away the blood on the floor. He put his wife's two travelling bags in the luggage compartment of his car and filled three garbage bags with new clothing she had bought for her trip, adding his own clothes which he had worn during the butchering. He drove to a local hardware store where he bought eighty feet of copper wire, then on to a dump where he burned the garbage bags. While there, he cut the wire into strips and bound the packages of grisly remains. That night, he dropped them into the river.

The next day, Kimberley and Elizabeth joined their father in a fruitless search for Anna. Perhaps, they thought, she had actually taken off for England. The Missing Persons Bureau had no information about her.

A week later, an angler dropped his line in the river and brought up a strange-looking parcel with copper binding. It contained the left foot of a human being. It was not long before the police divers brought up the rest of the packages. Police checked with William to see if he had received word about his missing wife. He hadn't, he said. They talked to the girls, who they said knew nothing of their mother's whereabouts.

Police decided to check up on the copper wire. A salesman in one of the hardware stores they visited remembered selling a quantity of wire to a male customer. Police, suspicious about William, played a long shot. They arranged another visit to his home and brought along the salesman posing as a policeman. The salesman didn't have to take a second look. William was indeed the man who had bought the wire.

William, charged with murder, offered no defence in court. He remained unmoved through the trial, even when forty-six pictures of his wife's dismembered body were shown to the jury. Even the skull with its gaping orifice didn't affect him.

He has functioned well in prison, having been moved, after four years, from maximum to medium security. He doesn't talk about Anna, only about his daughters, one of whom is married now, with a son, and the other who is employed in clerical work.

His case reflects the long-standing effects of controlled hostility. Anna, unaware of what she was doing, goaded her husband into a state of simmering rage. The brief remark, "You men are all..." precipitated her into sudden death, and him into a circumstanced state of amnesia.

William has come for psychiatric guidance frequently and, as time goes on, the tragic past becomes increasingly hidden among the more recent happenings in his life.

He will return to society soon and he will never show violence again. He will be passive, and even kindly. That two-second period of violence can never be reproduced because it took him twenty years to gather the ingredients that brought it about.

**Murder in the after years**

There are privileges and problems in this period. Graduation from the work force is not always welcome. Frustration, uncertainty, loneliness, bereavement, and resentment may cloud emotional and mental capabilities to produce degrees of behavioral change from passive withdrawal to extremes of irrational and impulsive acts.

In this context, criminality may be a reactive occurrence. Although aggression has long since passed its peak, anger and rage-filled states may develop, which produce assailable or homicidal acts.

Homicidal acts over fifty years of age are uncommon. Less than eight per cent of first and second degree murder charges involve this age group. Although criminality becomes infrequent and homicide is rare after age seventy, murder can be the result of a tangled web of erratic and bizzare circumstances. Such circumstances are usually found in family situations and stem from various stresses.

As aging itself is a slow evolution to senility, the mental, emotional and physical attributes of an individual slowly deteriorate, with changes in reasoning ability, effectiveness, and the ability to form normal judgments. In addition, there is the insidious appearance of an unhappy state known as "emotional apathy."

In a legal sense, there are many difficulties to overcome in order to give the older accused a fair trial. Such questions as intent to do a criminal act, appreciation of the consequences of the act, the mental competence and ability to know and understand trial procedures, and finally the flexibility to instruct counsel are some of the ongoing problems.

The aged person is not the mirror of normal man. Ignorance of geriatric inroads at trial may lead to an unfavorable bias on the part of the prosecution. The inability of an accused to remember, or even to give proper responses on examination, may be prejudicial to him. It may indeed be difficult for members of a jury panel to understand the motivations and actions of the aged mind.

I have taken great interest in this age group, in the belief that serious crime in the aged has to be evaluated very carefully, to ensure that the accused receives a just and fair hearing, a well-considered sentence and appropriate treatment.

Joseph is one of a numbe of people I have known who illustrates difficulties in this area. He was seventy-four in February of 1977 when he stabbed his sister-in-law, Betty to death and severely wounded his wife,Olive, for no apparent reason. He was a tall, slim, imposing man with a hearing aid, and the kind of figure you might see in an advertisement for a senior citizens' residence or club. With all due respect for his seniority in the community however, I have to say he was a demanding, irritating old codger who was always rubbing people the wrong way.

I saw him at the Quinte Regional Detention Centre forty-eight hours after the crime and at weekly intervals thereafter. I arranged a complete evaluation for him at the Clarke Institute of Psychiatry in Toronto, gave evidence at his trial for second degree murder, attended to him during his stay at Kingston Penitentiary, worked with his lawyer to obtain a retrial, and gave evidence when he finally won his new trial. The latter session ended with the jury finding him guilty of manslaughter.

Joseph was born of affluent parents and received his education at no fewer than three private schools. Employed by the postal service for forty years, he managed to find time to buy and sell diamonds and deal in used cars, accumulating considerable wealth along the way. He drove expensive cars and was known to have large sums of money with him wherever he went. But he was frugal and watched how every penny was spent – by him and his wife.

He was married three times and each marriage was fraught with serious emotional differences. His third effort, at age sixty, was full of ongoing disagreements because he insisted on controlling absolutely all household and personal purchases, including the buying of groceries and clothes, and the investment of both his and his wife's income. His autocratic, demanding, closed mind eventually caused spouse number three, Olive, to leave him and go live with her sister, Betty.

Olive's decision was totally incomprehensible to him. He just did not understand why she would leave him. He had, after all, done everything he could to ensure the economic well-being of the marriage. It was the approach of Valentine's Day that prompted him to try to get his wife back. He invited both Olive and Betty to the house and they agreed to come.

This is what Joseph told me in our first interview:

"I bought two boxes of Valentine chocolates and made a pot of coffee. When the girls came in, I invited them into the kitchen for coffee and asked my wife to talk to me. Instead, they started laughing and mocking and eating my chocolates. That's all I remember until a policeman stuck his head around the door and asked, 'What's going on?' Betty was lying on the floor. I had hold of my wife's wrists and she was yelling, 'Betty, Betty?' I didn't know what had happened."

What had happened was that he had murdered his sister-in-law, and very nearly murdered his wife, by stabbing them repeatedly with a kitchen knife. It had been a veritable bloody orgy.

And he remembered nothing about any of it.

Over the next two months, Joseph was very demanding. He wanted to be given bail, and repeated the request over and over. He was frequently on sick parade, complaining of various ailments, and showed little interest, or even awareness, of the seriousness of the charge against him. He couldn't understand why his case wasn't being considered immediately and kept reminding custodial people that he had to return home to plant the thirty-two tulip bulbs he had put in a plastic bag under the stairs.

He was talkative and reminisced often about his career and his shrewd business deals. There was no mention of remorse in connection with the death of Betty, nor did he display any interest in the condition of his wife. Instead, he reviewed, over and over, the role Betty had played in the estrangement of Olive. It was she, he maintained, who had been at the root of all his problems.

At his first trial, Dr. Stephen Hucker, of the Clarke Institute, and I gave psychiatric evidence indicating our belief that the accused, at the time of the offence, had been in an irrational, confused state of mind, brought about by emotional frustration and magnified by a state of toxic confusion relating to ongoing pneumonia.

Our evidence didn't help him. The jury returned a verdict of guilty of murder in the second degree. And one juror declared, after adjournment, "Any old bugger that put thirty-two stab wounds into his wife and sister-in-law knew exactly what he was doing. He's guilty as hell – pneumonia or not."

At his second trial, old Joseph did nothing to endear himself to anyone. He had a hostile attitude that irritated the prosecution and his impersonal, uninvolved stance even annoyed his own lawyer. He gave the impression of an irritable, irascible old man, totally self-justifying and egocentric.

The jury, which also had little sympathy for him, brought in a verdict of guilty of manslaughter and the judge, taking into account the fact that he had already served some twenty-six months in custody, gave him a six-year sentence.

Joseph, grumbling and snorting, has now been released to parole authorities. He is presently living with old friends who have taken on the responsibility for his care and supervision for the remaining years of his life.

* * *

Only a few people enter the rim of senility, as intercurrent infections, malignancies and degenerative illnesses kill them before their natural time. However, there are serious problems in store for aged people, long before there is any question of senility.

People over seventy may still manage to display some of the sparkle of their old lifestyles, but they soon become aware of a decrease in their physical abilities and their potential for really enjoying life as they once did. They also become increasingly aware that life has passed them by – and the world is too busy to have noticed.

The mental picture of the senior citizen in our youth-oriented society, conjures up glowing associations like the "Golden Years" and the "Sunshine Years." What superlatives! What garbage! No words can really describe the experience of aging. The aged person is an alien in his own society, a person with a different lifestyle, with altered emotional responses, who has withdrawn behind the curtain of today to muse idly about years gone by.

Society shuns the different personality. The defective, the eccentric, the disabled, the aged – all are of little account really, because they are not useful to the economic and social segments of our culture.

There are some genetically strong, resourceful old people, and there is a percentage of aged individuals whose life characteristics have been warped by bias, selfishness, hostility and other mental and emotional afflictions. The laws of senility through arterial alterations may produce personality changes, with poor memory, lessened controls and various kinds of erratic behavior.

As our aged population grows, so will the number of behavioral offences. Problems of assault, murder and suicide will increase in direct proportion to population numbers. They will pose special problems requiring special consideration in the courts so as to ensure justice.

Nobody would have thought that Harold would commit murder. Intelligent, quiet-spoken, confident, kindly, university-trained, he had risen to the level of senior executive in a large corporation in Toronto. He was one of those "pillars of society," someone who knew him said, a big businessman with a sense of corporate and civic responsibility.

Who would have thought he would kill his wife? Yet, in June of 1966, at age sixty-five, Harold entered Kingston Penitentiary to begin a life sentence for her murder. He had intended it to be murder-suicide but it didn't work out that way. She had died. He hadn't.

In penitentiary, I identified his psychiatric state as an endogenous mental depression. My first interview revealed considerable depth to his depression which, I concluded, had affected his evidence at trial.

Harold described his feeling before the murder as one of complete hopelessness. He had a "very definite feeling," he stated, that he had had enough of life and wanted to die.

After the murder, he refused to call a lawyer because he saw no point to it. He had tried to end his life and failed. Now, he just wanted to cut his throat. Later he did agree to have a lawyer, though he was cautious not to divulge too much information about himself. He didn't tell the lawyer, for instance, that he had taken an overdose of pills the previous year.

"Because of my position in the community, they took me to the hospital and treated it as a heart attack," he told me. "That was it as far as the company, and outsiders, were concerned. My problem was that I took more than the lethal dose. I was disappointed to be alive."

When I started digging for reasons, he shrugged. "There was no incident that precipitated it. Can you understand what I'm saying? I just didn't want to live anymore."

In ensuing interviews, Harold laid bare his tangled emotional life, which began at age twenty-four when he married a French student with what he called an "inordinate streak of jealousy." The marriage produced eleven years of chaotic, explosive and unhappy experiences which terminated in divorce. Five years later, he remarried. He was a heavy drinker and his second wife became alcohol-dependent. Within three years their marriage was in a state of complete deterioration.

By way of complicating his life, he fell in love with a third woman. It was completely by accident, he maintained. He hadn't been looking for anyone. It had been the last thing on his mind. But it had happened. He became aware of a deterioration in his life and developed a very strong dependency on sleeping pills and alcohol.

He became more reflective as our interviews continued:

"If anybody had tried to tell me I was an alcoholic, or that I was not normal mentally, I would not have believed them. But looking back, I know I had not been thinking rationally for a long time."

This is what he had to say about the day of the murder:

"I'm not sure I intended to kill her. I intended as much as you can use the word 'intend' after you sit and drink for three hours steadily. I just got up and said, 'The hell with it.' And that was it."

He went into the garage adjoining the house, fitted a long length of garden hose to the exhaust of the car and pulled it into the room in which his wife sat, unaware of what he was doing. Then he started the engine of the car. The carbon monoxide did the rest.

Some months after being admitted to K.P., he was treated with a series of electroshocks. His reaction to treatment was dramatic. He became the bright, intellectual, affable person he remembered being in earlier years.

These are his words:

"My state of mind changed with shock treatments. I accepted my new life and forgot the old one."

Harold hadn't been cut out for the kind of work he was doing. He would have been happier living a more physical life, perhaps in some rugged climate. His life as a business executive oppressed his individuality and destroyed his capacity for human warmth and kindness. The petty differences of everyday living frustrated him and he developed into an unhappy, selfish man, hunting for answers that simply were not to be found in his lifestyle. In prison, he managed to rediscover his original self – a warm, caring and unsophisticated man.

He was released on parole after serving ten years and today is functioning satisfactorily in society at the venerable age of eighty. At K.P., everyone remembers him kindly. Affable, always considerate, he won the respect of the custodial staff and of many inmates as well.

Harold had been assigned to the psychiatric ward as an orderly and I'll always remember the big smile that crept into his face the afternoon fellow orderlies gathered to wish him a happy sixty-seventh birthday. They had chipped in and bought him a pipe and a tin of tobacco and someone in the kitchen, ignoring the prohibition against such things, had made him a cake.

It was the first birthday any of us had ever celebrated in the joint.

**CHAPTER 11**

# Insanity Pleas

Canadian law provides for specific courses of action when a plea of insanity is under consideration in court. By way of a Warrant Of Remand, for example, a judge may send an accused person to a mental hospital for psychiatric evaluation for a period not exceeding sixty days. If a person is found to have been insane at the time of his offence, a warrant signed by the Lieutenant-Governor of the province of jurisdiction confines him to a hospital for the criminally insane until such time as the yearly Board of Review of that province finds him sufficiently well to return to society under a supervisory parole.

The law is specific enough, yet there are paradoxes.

Take, for instance, the Lieutenant-Governor's warrant of committal. I know two individuals who, on the Review Board's recommendation, left a mental hospital on probation, returned to society and committed another crime. In both cases, the second offence was committed under circumstances indicating the person was well mentally. This means an individual may arrive in prison on a sentence for robbery, and still be under a warrant for an offence he committed perhaps ten or fifteen years earlier, while he was mentally ill.

Lawyers are reluctant in minor cases to expose clients to a long, indefinite sentence resulting from acknowledged insanity, knowing that a simple guilty plea may result in a much shorter sentence. The effect of this is that our prisons have a number of inmates serving terms as sane people when, in fact, they are mentally deranged.

The paradoxes can cause considerable confusion.

How is it that a man, who is considered to be insane at the time he commits a bank holdup, can be deemed sane when he steps out of that bank into the street and shoots a policeman?

Again, how is it that an individual who is known to have been insane when he committed a murder can be tried and convicted as a sane person simply because he won't enter an insanity plea?

The issue of pleading insanity before the courts is one of prime importance to the psychiatrist, particularly so if the psychiatrist involved is working inside a penitentiary. The issue, however, needs some historical perspective and this I'll try to provide here.

* * *

In the normal mind, mood, perception, memory, reason, judgment, insight and intelligence are integrated functions. In abnormal minds, there is dysfunction in these areas. A serious mood disorder, for example, is always a component of manic-depressive illness. Disorders of perception, such as hallucinations, are consistent components of schizophrenia and toxic delirium. Memory loss may be attendant in brain injury, drugs and alcohol overuse, and senile degeneration. Judgment suffers greatly in paranoid illness, wherein the person's conviction, though contrary to fact, controls his behavior. Lack of reasoning and the inability to comprehend, is a common denominator in many mental illnesses. It is a process which depends on perception and memory to formulate solutions to new experiences. Judgment is the ability to correctly evaluate situations of varying complicity by discerning and comparing.

Legal insanity is based on a strict formula drawn from select areas of mental function: intelligence; judgment, wherein fixed delusions may develop; and reason, which can become blunted so that the person cannot understand, appreciate or predict the outcome of his acts. Memory may be temporarily destroyed, thus affording the person diminished ability to use his past experiences to weigh facts and determine rightness and wrongness.

The law as it relates to insanity goes back to the days of the great English lawyer, Sir Edward Coke, who, in 1628, established the following:

"A man can have no felonious intent and therefore cannot be convicted of it if he is so deprived of his reason that he resembles an animal rather than a man.

"Where a person of sound memory and discretion unlawfully killeth any reasonable creature with malice aforethought, either expressed or implied, he will be brought under the king's peace for trial."

Some one hundred years later, Sir Matthew Hale, Lord Chief Justice of England ruled:

"If a man of sound mind commits a crime, he cannot be tried if he becomes insane, and if he becomes insane after the trial, he cannot be punished."

The James Hadfield case provided a further evolution in law. On May 15, 1800, he fired his pistol at King George the Third from the pit of London's Drury Lane Theatre. He missed his target and was immediately overpowered and removed. The king and his son, the Duke of York, later questioned him and discovered that he had been in the army and had once been the duke's batman.

Subsequent investigation revealed that Hadfield had received serious head wounds in battle and these had affected his reasoning. His friends and associates noted that, since his injury, he had become moody, preoccupied and seclusive. Hadfield had indeed become strange. He imagined he had constant contact with God, that the world was coming to an end and that he was to sacrifice himself for instant salvation. He thought he should become a blessed sacrifice. Under the delusion of still being in battle, he convinced himself that if he were shot and killed in war, it wouldn't have the same value as if he had sacrificed himself by committing suicide.

Hadfield was brought to trial for high treason. It was a trial that would go into the legal history books. He was defended by a lawyer named Thomas Erskine, who established that he was suffering from compelling and overpowering delusions, and who explained that people with these extreme delusions could conceal them so effectively, that individuals of intelligence could be deceived into regarding them as normal.

James Hadfield was declared not guilty because he was "under the influence of insanity at the time the act was committed." The case established the legal precedent of insane delusions, making it possible to use them as defence for murder.

The legal controversy then focussed around the moral issue of rightness and wrongness, and the belief that a person, who knows he is doing something wrong, is accountable for his actions. In 1812, an able and widely-known businessman, who had extensive trade connections with Russia, shot and killed then British Prime Minister Spencer Percival in the House of Commons. The assailant, a man named Bellingham, claimed he had suffered numerous business losses due to the wars of the time and said the British Parliament was responsible for his problems. Specifically, he regarded Percival as the source of his misfortune.

Five days after the killing, Bellingham was brought to trial in London's famous Old Bailey courthouse. Lawyers entered a plea of insanity and requested a delay so that inquiries could be made in Liverpool concerning his previous behavior. Bellingham himself denied that he was insane and said he had committed his act to punish the prime minister. The judge, impelled by popular sentiment, refused the delay and ordered that the trial proceed. The jury returned a guilty verdict and he was hanged.

Evidence came later that Bellingham had been suffering from a kind of mania that prevented him from appreciating the difference between right and wrong. His case was one of the main turning points in legal philosophy and brought new attention to the whole question of insanity and the law.

Perhaps the most famous case in this area is that of a Glasgow Scotsman named Daniel McNaughton who, in 1834, shot and killed Edward Drummond, private secretary to Prime Minister Sir Robert Peel. Drummond was shot in the mistaken belief that he was the prime minister.

"The whole question will turn upon this," prosecutor Sir William Webb Follett said at the trial. "If you believe the prisoner, at the time he committed this act, was not a responsible agent, if you believe that when he fired the pistol he was incapable of distinguishing between right and wrong, if you believe that he was under the influence or control of disease of the mind which prevented him from being conscious that he was committing a crime, if you believe that he did not know he was violating the law, then definitely he is entitled to your acquittal. But it is my duty to tell you that nothing short of that will excuse him upon the principle of English law.

"Excuse him that he had a morbid delusion upon some subject which could not exist in a wholly sane person, this is not enough. If he had the degree of insight which enabled him to know and distinguish between right and wrong, if he knew what could be the effects of the crime and consciously committed it, and if with that consciousness he wilfully committed it, he gentlemen, is not excused from punishment."

McNaughton's defence counsel, Arthur Cockburn, Q.C., argued that the right and wrong test had no application in cases of delusion, because a person so affected cannot use good judgment in his conduct and therefore is in a state of mental aberration in which he is not criminally answerable for his actions.

Cockburn's concluding statement was a legal masterpiece. He said, "Proceeding as it does on a false case of conjecture of his own fancy, his judgment of right or wrong, responsibility that should attend it, is truly the same as none at all."

Cockburn proved that McNaughton, over the ten years of his life prior to the offence, had been harassed by terrible images, conjured up by his distorted mind. The accused felt he was being pursued by forces intent on destroying him. Cockburn followed the history of his client's travels in England, France and Italy. McNaughton was continually trying to get away from the people he suspected were following him. "I can get no rest from them, day or night," he said in a statement read in court. "They have accused me of crimes of which I am not guilty."

McNaughton was found not guilty by virtue of insanity and committed to a mental hospital. A panel of judges later formulated a law concerning crimes committed by persons afflicted with insane delusions.

It was a law which was to become one of the major instruments of justice: The McNaughton Rule. It is the functional rule in insanity cases in England and has been accepted as such in most English-speaking countries. In Canadian law, it forms part of the Criminal Code:

"No person shall be convicted of an offence in respect of an act or omission on his part while he was insane."

For the purpose of this section, a person is insane when he is in a state of natural imbecility, or has disease of the mind to an extent that renders him incapable of appreciating the nature and quality of an act or omission, or of knowing that an act or omission is wrong.

A person who has specific delusions, but is in other respects sane, shall not be acquitted on the ground of insanity unless the delusions caused him to believe in the existence of things that, if they existed, would have justified or excused his act or omission.

Everyone shall be presumed to be sane, and to have been sane, until the contrary is proved.

We have come a long way in the struggle to gain recognition in the courts of the fact of insanity. We have been able to demonstrate the effectiveness of legal instruments such as our warrants of committal and remand. And we are using them to good advantage.

My late friend, Dr. Kenneth McKnight, who at different times served the Ontario Hospital at Penetang and the Clarke Institute of Psychiatry in Toronto, provided some interesting statistics in support of the remands some years ago. In a study of one hundred accused persons remanded for psychiatric evaluation, fifty-five were found unfit to stand trial, and twenty-seven were eventually found not guilty because of insanity and committed to hospital under a Lieutenant Governor's warrant. The other eighteen were found to be mentally competent and sent to trial.

Dr. McKnight's extensive studies produced this profile of the mentally deranged murderer:

(a) He is between thirty and thirty-four years of age.
(b) He generally murders his victim in March.
(c) He usually kills on Tuesday.

Sixty-six per cent of victims were killed in their homes. In forty-one per cent of cases, they were shot; in fifteen per cent, stabbed; and in six per cent, strangled. The others died under various circumstances.

The question of an individual's mental state is an involved one which can take up a great deal of time in court. The complexity of the insanity plea is further intensified by the changing picture of the competency of the accused in standing trial. In some cases, the trial judge may insist on psychiatric testimony each morning to determine if the accused is mentally fit to stand trial that particular day. The competency of an

# Reward City

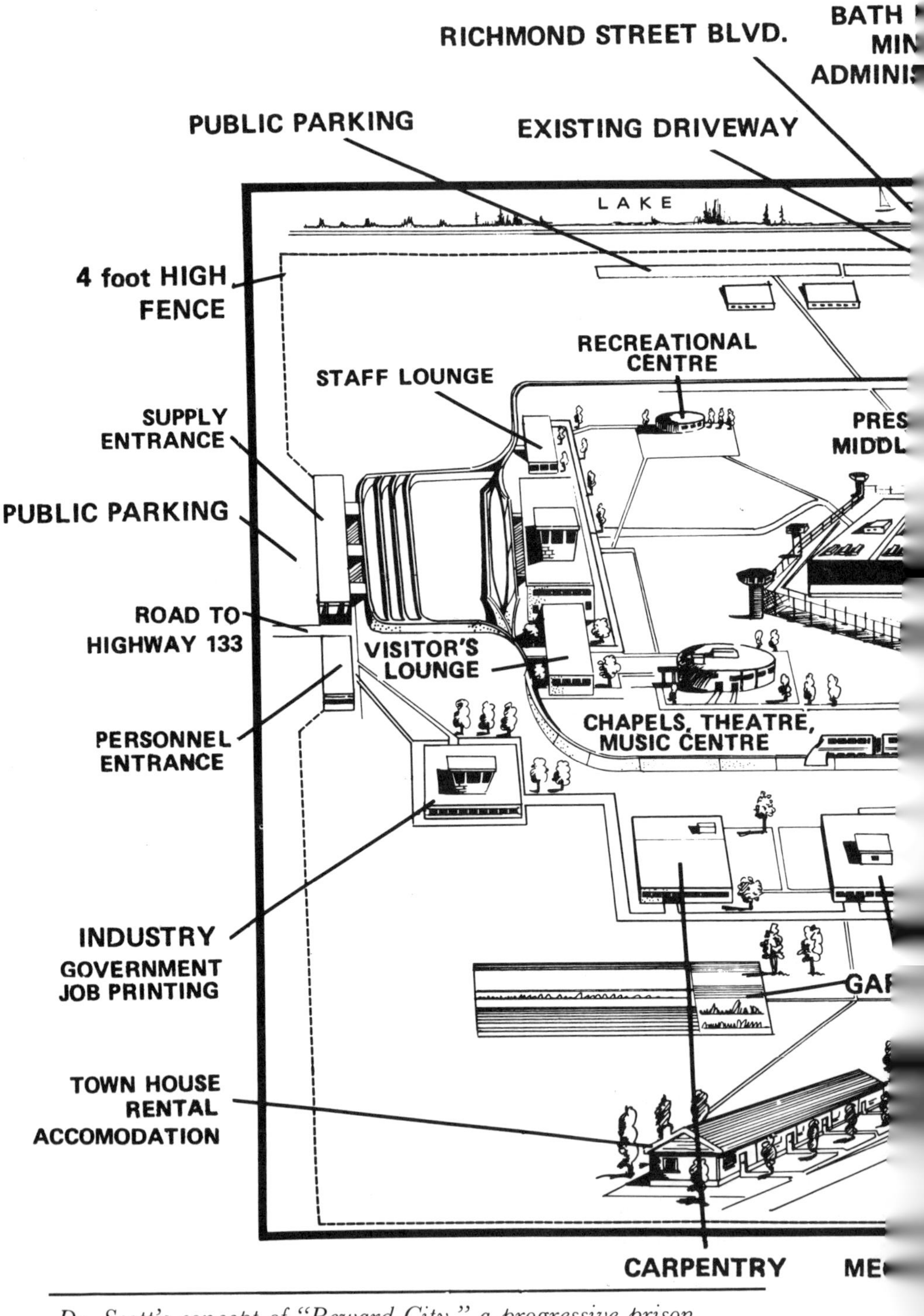


*Dr. Scott's concept of "Reward City," a progressive prison program.*
*(See Chapter 23)*

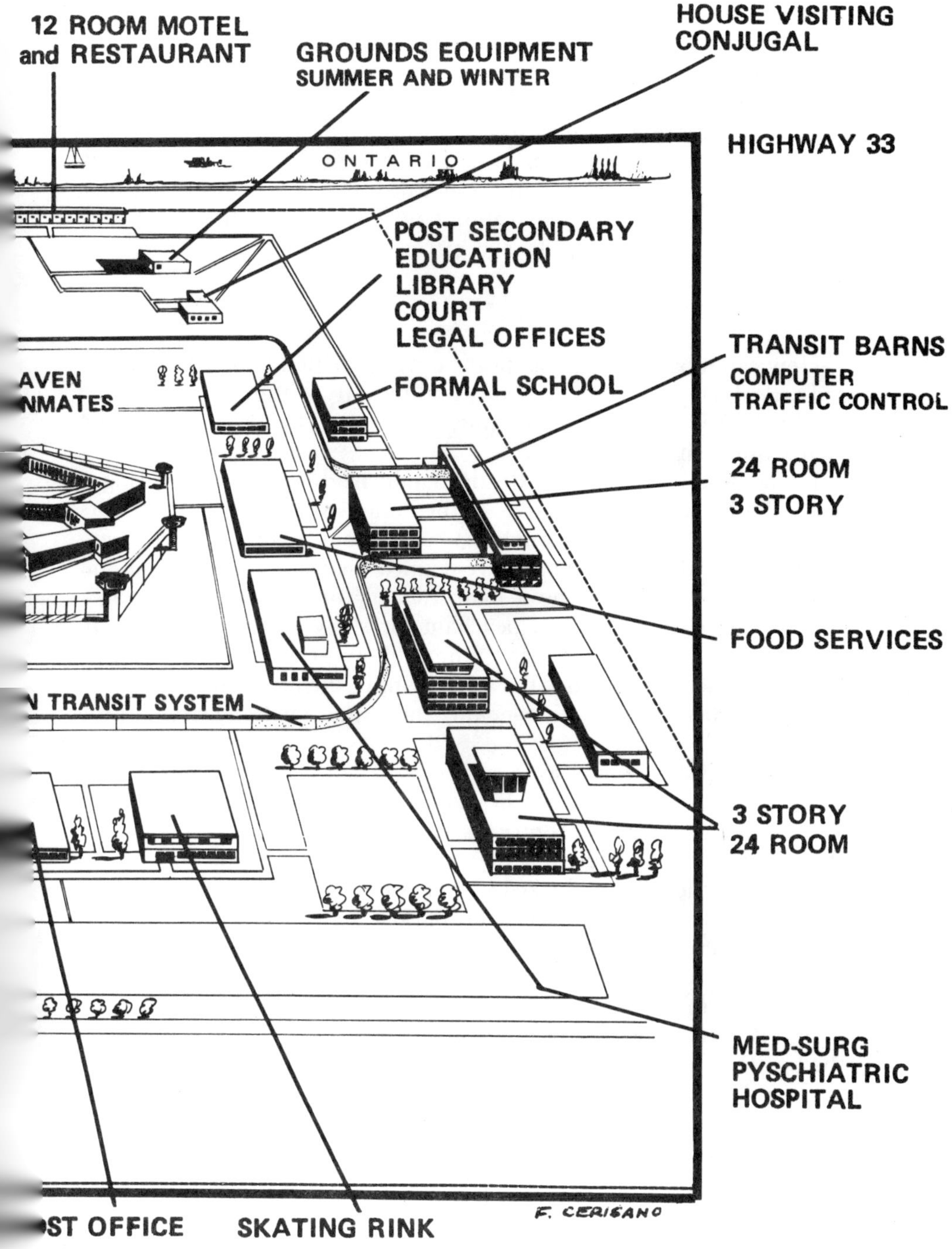
12 ROOM MOTEL
and RESTAURANT
GROUNDS EQUIPMENT
SUMMER AND WINTER
HOUSE VISITING
CONJUGAL
HIGHWAY 33
ONTARIO
POST SECONDARY
EDUCATION
LIBRARY
COURT
LEGAL OFFICES
TRANSIT BARNS
COMPUTER
TRAFFIC CONTROL
AVEN
NMATES
FORMAL SCHOOL
24 ROOM
3 STORY
FOOD SERVICES
N TRANSIT SYSTEM
3 STORY
24 ROOM
MED-SURG
PYSCHIATRIC
HOSPITAL
ST OFFICE
SKATING RINK
F. CERISANO

accused to stand trial involves his ability to comprehend the significance of the charges, to instruct his counsel in matters relating to the alleged offence, and to understand the court's purposes and procedures.

The psychiatrist appears in court as an expert witness. He gives evidence concerning the state of mind of the accused prior to and at the time of the offence, his ability to know right from wrong and his awareness of the consequences of his acts. I have been involved in numerous criminal cases in which insanity is pleaded and I can assure you that a great deal of care and preparation have gone into each.

And still we have these strange, paradoxical situations.

* * *

How can a bank robber be insane during the first half of his offence and sane during the second? Sanity and insanity within minutes of one another? The case of Toronto's much publicized "Beatle Bandit" posed such a question.

He became known as the Beatle Bandit because he was wearing a wig fashioned after the hairstyle of the famous singing group when he was arrested. Actually, he could also have become known as the "Santa Claus Bandit" because he had once donned the traditional red suit and flowing white beard during a bank robbery in Hamilton. He was a flamboyant character with a penchant for show and play-acting. He would literally burst into a bank, jump up on a counter, wave his gun in the air and demand that the tellers empty their cash drawers. The tellers, terrified by the weird-looking individual towering above them, never argued.

His first two hold-ups were successful. His third was a fiasco.

He was twenty-eight when he did his counter-climbing, gun-slinger routine at the Bank of Montreal's Downsview branch in Toronto in the fall of 1965, and this time he carried a 30 mm carbine. The tellers obeyed his orders and it looked like another successful robbery – until he got into his car, which he had parked just outside, and found it wouldn't start. As luck would have it, an off-duty detective named Jack Blanco was passing by the bank. Seeing the commotion, he stopped. In the meantime, the bank manager had come out onto the sidewalk with a gun. Blanco, an expert marksman, asked him for the weapon. When the Beatle Bandit got out of the car, he faced the armed detective, opened fire and hit him between the eyes. Blanco died almost immediately.

The bandit was subsequently brought to trial on a charge of first degree murder, convicted and sentenced to be hanged. His sentence was later commuted to one of life imprisonment.

He was an intense, much-disturbed man when he came to see me in the psychiatric office at Kingston Penitentiary. He spoke in a serious, hushed voice and his words didn't come easily.

"Doc, I got this ticking in my head."

He tapped his forehead with his fingers and closed his eyes, as though the very act of touching his head was painful.

"I don't know if you can do anything, Doc, but I got this strange clock in my head, and it's beating faster all the time."

He paused. Not wanting to interrupt his train of thought, I decided to remain silent.

"The clock's ticking all the time. I don't understand it. The ticks come so fast and so close together. They're driving me crazy. I haven't slept more than two hours a night since I got here. I can't take it. You've got to help me."

He described the ticks as being somewhat like stabbing electrical charges. He had been suffering from them a long time, he said.

In my professional experience, this was a very unusual condition. I established in the interview that he suffered from a serious mental condition in which his relation with reality had been altered by the messages given to his mind by the mechanical ticks. It was an ongoing hallucinatory experience. His general file, however, revealed no diagnosis of a psychiatric disability and no evidence of any psychiatric representation having been made at his trial.

I advised him that I would admit him to the psychiatric unit as soon as a bed became available. He never made it to the unit. The morning after our interview, guards found him dead in his cell. He had severed the femoral arteries in his groin and died quietly on his cot.

After his death, the intensity of his words bothered me. I began to wonder if, somehow, I had missed something in the interview. I called the Metropolitan Toronto Police, the lawyer who defended him and the lawyer who prosecuted the case. From their information, I was able to piece together a strange human jigsaw picture.

The Beatle Bandit had been a social malcontent for two years prior to his last robbery – and an unbalanced social malcontent in every respect. He had grandiose schemes which he discussed freely with astounded friends and acquaintances. He was destined, he told them, to set up a military government and rule Canada. In conversation with his lawyer, he confided that he had stashed away at home the money he had stolen. It was to be used to buy weapons and pay his followers for their loyalty.

Investigating detectives who visited his apartment found an interesting collection of things. They found a rack of six automatic rifles, eight hundred rounds of ammunition and a room full of posters with revolutionary print-outs. They also found several orderly piles of bills totalling $36,000.

Of particular interest to me was the fact that both defending and prosecuting lawyers considered that the bandit had been mentally ill for several years and that legally he was insane at the time of the robbery. He had, they said, labored under the delusionary belief that he was to lead Canada as head of a military government, and had committed the robbery as a consequence of his delusion.

His history of insane behavior, however, was technically wiped out when he stepped out of the bank. On the street, facing an armed opponent, he had drawn his gun, thus acknowledging that he was aware of the consequences of his action.

The Beatle Bandit's story is a strange one. He lived a serious and planned existence, controlled by his distorted mental beliefs. His suicide may have developed out of the tick messages in his brain, although we have no substantiation for this. I am confident, however, that he was unaware of the subtle legal lines that separated the stages of his offence, and that by stepping out of the bank, he had crossed over from his insane delusional world into the hapless world of sanity.

* * *

The case of Martin is one of the really strange examples of legal paradox, involving the question of whether a man is well enough to understand that he's pleading insanity.

Martin was a slim, trim, middle-aged professional man of proud bearing and dignified manner. However, that October day in 1973, when he came to see me in the psychiatric office at Joyceville Institution, he was in a very unhappy frame of mind. His blue eyes were moist with tears, his facial expression was tense, drawn and controlled, and his hands were clasped together tightly.

He had killed his wife the previous summer and had been given a life sentence for non-capital murder. He was going through those traumatic first months of prison existence when I first saw him. I can still hear him uttering the words, "Doctor help me. I'm a sick man. My thoughts are destroying my mind. I didn't kill my wife. It was a terrible accident. I'm sick. I'm being tortured. Save me, please. Please. I can't go on this way."

He continued without interruption. The words flowed like lava from a volcano.

"I've written letters to my friends. I've tried to explain. Doctor, I'm in hell. Please get me out. I can't kill myself because my soul will not permit me to die in jail."

There is part of my mind that I reserve for doubt and suspicion and there, in that little recess, I considered his behavior and concluded that he was not play-acting or trying to manipulate me. This, I determined, was a serious psychiatric emergency requiring immediate observation.

Martin was admitted to the Regional Psychiatric Centre where he remained for six months. There, he was totally occupied with his own welfare, wrote threatening and vindictive letters to people on the outside (among them his trial judge), and made frequent and unreasonable demands on the staff. It was a condition of martyred self-condemnation. He was full of self-pity, felt he was persecuted and wallowed in depression. In addition, he had no remorse over the death of his wife.

I decided to dig deeper into the case and contacted the lawyer who defended Martin and the one who prosecuted him. I also spoke to the psychiatrist who testified at his trial. Martin I learned, had been suffering from mental illness for more than a year prior to the offence but refused to allow his lawyer to enter a plea of insanity on his behalf. The prosecution was aware of Martin's condition but could do nothing. As the law now stands, only the defence can raise the insanity plea.

Martin had a great many staunch friends and associates in the business and professional world and they sent me numerous testimonials over the months. Some of them were very touching.

One correspondent wrote:

"The impression he left me with was of a sensitive, somewhat shy but friendly, honest, deeply religious man, greatly concerned with the welfare of people, possessed of a strong sense of social justice, one who holds strong views against hypocrisy, trite and humbug, whether in politics, religion or social relationships."

Another told the story aptly and in very few words:

"A shot was fired by a Great Champion, distracted and deranged."

In 1974, I reviewed the psychiatric story of this "Great Champion" with Arthur Maloney, Q.C., in Toronto. He was considering an appeal to the Supreme Court of Canada but there was a problem. Would Martin agree to go along with a revised plea – of insanity? I hurried back to Kingston and obtained his written word that he would concur with this plea. Then another problem arose. Was he well enough to understand his undertaking and give knowledgeable consent?

It was a strange situation. Martin was an insane person who had been convicted as sane. Now, as a legally sane individual, he was asking to be declared insane. I sat down with him in prison and explained the implications of his undertaking. If his insanity plea was accepted, I pointed out, he would be confined in a mental hospital under a Lieutenant-Governor's warrant. He would be there, I emphasized, for an indefinite period of time. I had to be sure he understood this. He did.

Martin was finally declared insane and sent to the Mental Health

Centre, Penetang, where he received extensive care and treatment. Then in mid-1977, with the approval of the Review Board, he was released. Today, he is trying to put the pieces of his life back together – and succeeding.

This case is unique in its history because the accused labored under the false belief that he was sane. This one lone man commanded the attention of the courts, the penitentiary psychiatrist services and, with the consistent write-in support of friends, saw his case reach the Supreme Court of Canada. In agreeing to pursue the course suggested to him, he revoked his sanity, accepted his illness, took treatment, and now has regained the treasured possession of all sane people – freedom.

**CHAPTER 12**

# Psychiatry in Court

Man is free to elect his degree of criminality, someone once said. This is true. It is also true that man is unable to determine his state of mind. And his state of mind is what, to a great extent, determines the way he does his time when he is in prison.

Mental health statistics indicate that ten per cent of the population suffer from a definable mental illness at some point during a lifetime. Five per cent suffer a disabling mental illness during a life span.

In federal penitentiaries, five per cent of the inmates suffer serious mental conditions. Of these, two per cent have had a clear-cut mental illness before going to prison. Two of every one hundred inmates commit offences which can be traced back, in some way, to their illness.

And that brings me to a problem that has bugged me for a long time. Bugged me? That's putting it mildly. It makes me hopping mad. I'm referring to the psychiatric nonsense that goes on all too often when an individual is brought into court to face criminal charges.

I am a psychiatrist and I have to say that I am very disturbed on occasion by the remarks of court psychiatrists, some of who display a sad lack of insight when dealing with someone with a mental problem.

What I'm saying is that I don't like it when someone gets screwed up by psychiatry. And, believe me, it happens.

Let me explain.

At times, psychiatric evidence in court may indicate a serious degree of mental illness that does not amount to insanity. In these cases, a sentence is sometimes determined on the basis of an estimate of time needed to treat the illness. Lawyers occasionally place great emphasis on the treatability of clients and this kind of evidence can cause no end of confusion. Confusion – and consternation on the part of the offender who may find himself up the prison creek for a lot longer than necessary.

I recall one case in which a judge handed down a twenty-eight-year sentence with a mandatory order for psychiatric treatment during that time. I can cite a number of similar situations. For example, I know an eighteen-year-old who received a life sentence, with a twenty-year minimum, because the psychiatric evidence postulated that that was the amount of time needed to treat the patient and make him non-dangerous to the public.

I treated both of these inmates and, after eight years of incarceration, judged them to be completely well. Yet they cannot be released. They cannot be freed because psychiatrists, in their blissful ignorance, estimated an overly long number of years for treatment and the judges concerned based their sentences on these false estimates.

It's alarming, because some of these opinions by court psychiatrists are made in the wake of an appalling lack of evidence. Some psychiatrists, with only hearsay knowledge of the real dynamics of mental illness in the younger age group, thus may add years to the sentence – and to the problems and frustrations – of the offender.

I am convinced that sentencing based on psychiatric predictions is wholly unfair and unjust. I believe, too, that some bright inmate of the future will appeal his case, basing it on the argument of faulty sentencing. I would be most anxious to hear the outcome.

There was a case of rape, heard in the Supreme Court of Ontario in September of 1972, in which the accused was a very prominent sportsman and proprietor of a retail sporting goods store. He was found guilty on two charges of indecent assault and one of rape and sentenced to life imprisonment.

James was twenty-eight, and had no previous criminal record. He had had a conspicuous sports record in school and was later very active in hockey and baseball organizations. He was an amiable, highly sociable individual who, in 1970, had received a citizen's award for sportsman-of-the-year.

His arrest shocked his home town and his trial was the sensation of the whole surrounding area. It was no wonder. Everybody knew him – and everybody admired him. Up until then, anyway.

His offences occurred on two consecutive nights and involved two girls in their mid-teens, whom he accosted in a quiet suburban area. One of the girls accepted his sexual advances in a passive way, the other fought him off. He was arrested two weeks later when he committed an indecent assault on another female. Much to his surprise, she turned out to be a policewoman, assigned as a decoy to trap the rapist.

He was found guilty on all charges and two psychiatrists testified at the time of sentencing that he suffered from an "aggressive psychopathic personality". It was an incurable condition, they said. It would take at least twenty years for his sexually aggressive characteristics to disappear. On the basis of the psychiatric testimony, he was sentenced to life.

James entered Kingston Penitentiary as a rapist and child molestor.

He was met with taunts, blows and rejection, and lived in fear of physical abuse. After one particularly savage beating, he was transferred to Millhaven Institution for his own protection.

I saw him regularly in consultation there and had the opportunity to check every aspect of his institutional existence – his work, recreation and activities on his range. It was my opinion that he was not an aggressive psychopathic personality. Though he was skilled in evading issues, he was not aggressive and had none of the indifference, apathy and callousness found in the classical psychopath. He formed friendships with some inmates and learned the prison's low-profile "mind your own business" attitude. After three years of ongoing visits, I could find no evidence whatsoever, in any context, of the malignant symptom of the psychopathic personality.

James had kept in contact with his trial counsel and had been put in touch with an appeal lawyer in Toronto. His hope was that he would be able to appeal his case on grounds that there may have been errors in the court's handling of it. I wrote the lawyer suggesting that the case be appealed on other grounds – namely that the diagnosis of a psychopathic personality, an aggressive type, was faulty and that he, the appellant, was, in effect, not psychopathic. I explained that he had been the victim of overwhelming stresses prior to the offences and these had triggered his angry outbursts, which he had directed at females.

I had done my homework. I had five years of clinical proof to back up my diagnosis. I knew James very well by now, better I'm sure than a lot of people. I had studied him, analyzed him, and explored his family background from childhood on.

James's basic problem had to do, quite simply, with women. His mother was very domineering and his two sisters were older than he and tended to boss him around. His wife was an autocratic person who treated him like a child whenever there was a family row, which was often. Just prior to the offences, there had been a serious argument and she had left for Florida. This had angered him.

It was stress that had sparked his anger and it was his life's experience with women that made him turn this anger on those two hapless girls.

In a letter to the Ontario Court of Appeal, I explained that James's personality lacked the hostility frequently seen in the serious sex offender, and that his amenability to treatment had been positive. I added, "The appellant's personality exhibits features of immaturity but psychiatric assessment in the penitentiary does not confirm the diagnosis that the appellant suffers from a mental illness or a character disorder."

The Appeal Court reviewed the case and unanimously reduced the sentence from life to fifteen years. In 1980, James was released.

He is presently functioning well in society under the careful and supportive supervision of his parole officer.

The value of psychiatric evidence in criminal cases has been proven many times. Expert opinions are sought by both defence and prosecuting lawyers. Each takes the evidence of the expert and attempts to use it to suit his particular cause. There are, however, a number of inherent dangers here.

Frequently, psychiatrists use diagnostic terms like "aggressive anti-social personality," "psychopathic personality," "schizophrenia," or "paranoia." Unfortunately, these diagnoses carry mental pictures with them in the eyes of a an unsophisticated jury. Once such a diagnostic statement is made, the expert witness adds the characteristic symptomatology and applies it to the case at hand.

I have been to court as one of those expert witnesses many times and I don't mind saying that I get pretty upset when I see a psychiatrist becoming involved in carefully selected questions raised by the opposing counsel to establish his case.

Consider for a moment the following courtroom scenario:

Question: "And now Doctor, tell me about the mental state of the accused. You have stated that the accused suffered from a mental condition called schizophrenia, that his mind is disturbed, that he is moody and preoccupied. Is this a common mental disease?"

Answer: "Yes, it is one of the most common mental diseases."

Q: "Well now, does everyone with schizophrenia have criminal tendencies?"

A: "No."

Q: "And what percentage do have criminal tendencies?"

A: "A very small percentage."

Q: "Do you believe that the accused in the box suffers from a mild, or advanced, case of schizophrenia?"

A: "I believe he is in a moderately advanced state."

Q: "Does the accused, in your opinion, know he has done some act which is wrong? No, I'll phrase my question in a simpler way. Do you think that the accused in the box at this moment knows what is going on in court and why he is here?"

A: "Yes, I do."

Q: "Now tell me Doctor, is schizophrenia a treatable illness?"

A: "It depends on how long it has been established, how the patient cooperates and how effective the prescribed treatment is."

Q: "Do you believe that a schizophrenic loses his disease as a man loses his appendix – suddenly?"

A: "No, it takes a long time."

Q: "How long, in your opinion, would it take in the case of the accused at the bar to be treated so he would be safe in society?"

A: "A number of years."

Q: "You must be more definite in your answer. I'll help you. Under ten years. Between ten and twenty years. Over twenty years?"

A: "It depends upon the case."

Q: "Now Doctor, with your skill and expert knowledge, and your examination of the accused, what opinion would you give? You must have some idea."

A: "Probably between fifteen and twenty years."

This examination, although fair and straightforward enough, establishes for the crown that the accused, under average conditions, may take from fifteen to twenty years to modify or cure his symptoms. Obviously, the crown attorney is laying the basis for a sentence of considerable severity and the defence psychiatrist has given him all the invaluable evidence he needs to present to the jury.

In the following scenario, based on a case in which I was involved, the answers in the cross-examination exclude the matter of diagnosis.

Q: "Now Doctor, tell me about the mental state of the accused. You have stated that he has symptoms of a condition characterized by preoccupation with fantasy and that he has moody spells, shuns people, is very seclusive and, at times, misinterprets what people say to him. Has he, or has he not, a mental illness?"

A: "He has a degree of mental illness described as a disordered state of reality. His symptoms, and many other behavioral symptoms, are lumped together under the descriptive name of schizophrenia. The symptoms vary in intensity in relationship to the circumstances surrounding a person at any given time."

Q: "Does one with these symptoms have criminal tendencies?"

A: "Again, it depends on the case. For instance, if a person with these symptoms is ridiculed or rejected, angry reactions may develop in him, which could result in criminal acts."

Q: "Do you believe that the accused in the box suffers from a mild, or advanced, degree of schizophrenia?"

A: "I can't answer that question because the condition you mention is a fluctuating one which may have acute periods and dormant states. The latter states may last for months at a time and permit individuals to function satisfactorily at home and at work."

Q: "As a result of your study of the case, do you believe that the accused knows in retrospect that this court case is a result of his alleged wrongful act?"

A: "Yes, I do."

A: "Now Doctor, with your skill and experience, and your examination of the accused, what opinion would you give about the possibility of a cure in a condition of this nature?"

A: "I can't give you a definite answer. It depends upon the case."

From this examination, no inference can be drawn with regard to the time required for the man's condition to improve. By avoiding the diagnosis, I was in a better position to describe the case rather than the disease.

There was a look of frustration on the prosecutor's face as he sat down after the interrogation. He had figured, I think, on getting some more specific information. As it was, he couldn't recommend a sentence of years roughly equivalent to some preposterously estimated period of time for a cure.

I was content. Nobody was getting screwed up by psychiatry in this case.

**CHAPTER 13**

# Suicides, Slashings and Other Stories

A custodial officer I know came over to me one day as I stood in the middle of King Street, staring blankly at the massive gray walls of old Kingston Penitentiary, and jokingly asked me if I was thinking of buying the place. It was a fine old building indeed, he said, with a truly commanding view of Lake Ontario.

I don't remember what I answered. I think I joked back about trying to find the mortgage money, or something equally inane. I know I didn't tell him what I was really thinking about.

I do that sometimes. Stare at prisons, I mean. Not just at Kingston Penitentiary which is well, spectacular in a way, if you fancy old fortress-type structures, but even at places that don't really look like prisons. Places like Joyceville and Millhaven Institutions that look more like community colleges, for example.

When I leave these places, I go out through the gates, walk toward my car and then stop. I smell the air, listen to the sounds of traffic and passers-by and feel the freedom around me. Believe me, you can feel it, once you've been inside.

Then I turn around and look at the prison and wonder how many of the guys inside ever manage to make it when they are finally sprung.

As I look back over the years, I marvel at the strength and resistance of a person who can handle ten to twenty years in a penitentiary and return to society with even modest motivation and hope of finding a place for himself.

It may be true that prisons don't actually injure the minds of inmates but it is also true that they excise some of their personality and seldom replace it with anything else.

What develops inside the walls is a prison mind, a complex, often mysterious thinking instrument that conjures up all manner of ailments, real and imagined, and a complementary list of remedies, sometimes strange, often frightening.

People can talk all they want about the gourmet meals they supposedly serve up behind the walls, the color televisions and the expensive sports equipment, but I can tell you that prisons aren't really pleasant places. They turn people into robots. They force inmates into adopting formal, specific and regulated routines, unfamiliar to any normal life patterns. No prisoner ever accepts the loss of his freedom, his right to dress as he pleases, buy what he pleases – and, oh yes, the right to steal when he pleases.

It's a far cry from free society where a person has the right to choose his own destiny. Free man is not treasonable if he elects to lead a criminal life. If he is really successful, he may even opt to play it safe with the government and report his income, making sure, of course, that everything looks legitimate. In face, he may be just like any other citizen – except that he's a crook.

Quasi-criminal man moves all around us. A car dealer has arrangements with his clients allowing five hundred dollars more for a trade-in as long as the client pays half of it back to him under the table. A dentist maintains two sets of accounts, one for the income tax office, one for himself. A businessman buys materials for a construction job and reports losing some of it to truck thieves. The material ends up on the site of his new summer home.

It's a fact of life that most people aren't greatly concerned over an impaired driving charge, a supermarket theft, or a charge of possessing stolen goods – as long as their offence doesn't make the local newspaper. Such a quasi-criminal is, by definition, a person who has wage-earning resources which he supplements with acquisitive acts against society.

"Wouldn't you agree, sir," an inmate asked me one day, "that a great many thieves never see the inside of a prison?"

Of course, I had to agree. People involved in income tax fraud, for example, might well be caught but conviction might take the form of restitution and fine and the offender, who doesn't go to jail, remains a citizen rather than an inmate.

The inmate who figures that all is not fair in crime and punishment may have a point. After all, the criminal is the individual who is caught, convicted and sentenced to prison, and not the one who eludes the law, or who is apprehended but not incarcerated.

And so the inmate, cut off from the mainstream for a period of time, his movements curtailed by bars, his days punctuated by the clonking sounds of lock mechanisms, his nights lonely and barren, develops his prison mind.

"Hi man, how is your world?" I ask Number so-and-so who has come into my office for consultation.

And he just looks at me and says, "Shit man, I ain't got no world."

The prison psychiatrist functions in a brackish environment. He is never the master of his own decisions because his patients consider his actions and his counsel in relation to the overwhelming influence of the inmate code. In addition, the doctor's every decision is subject to the security directions of the institution.

The subculture labels a psychiatric patient a *bug*, a term denoting a lack of reliability, so inmates are cautious about being seen too often around the doctor's office. They are also careful of what they say when they do see the psychiatrist. They are often uncomfortable in describing their institutional conflicts and will never mention other inmates even though their problems may revolve around them. Sometimes, they become hostile.

"Don't play head games."

"Stop screwing up my head."

I have had both admonitions thrown at me. Many inmates reject outright the emotionally threatening effects of the skilled therapist as dangerous and manipulative. Only a few inmates will consciously waive their inmate loyalties and seriously embark upon a therapeutic program.

More often than not, an inmate's request for psychiatric consultation is based on his need for sedative medication, his wish for a transfer to another range or his desire to change his prison employment. The request is often made in a veiled, demanding way, with the implication that if it is refused, there may be serious consequences. Suicide, self-mutilation and the swallowing of foreign objects are common bargaining devices.

So is hostage-taking. I am reminded of that every now and then when I have in my office a hostile inmate who refuses to sit down, or who wears a big coat. I say to myself, "this man could pull a knife and..." I don't dwell on such thoughts but I often wonder how my civilian counterpart, comfortably ensconced in a quietly elegant office and caring for a well-heeled clientele of peacefully unhappy souls, would react in such a situation.

Inmates use other means of bargaining too. They sometimes refuse to work, go on hunger strikes, demand segregation from the population, show up on sick parade for nuisance value, set fire to their cells, destroy property and write angry letters to members of Parliament, Penitentiary Service officials and the newspapers.

The penitentiary psychiatric services grant inmate requests for consultations and, of course, deal with referrals from the classification department, the psychologist, the institution discipline board and such groups as the Special Review Board.

The National Parole Service and local parole boards frequently ask for consultant advice on inmates with a history of unpredictable or dangerous behavior. Such an inmate, however, if competent, may refuse consultations and any prescribed medical care, including hospitalization, tests and examinations, except when these are mandatory under law, or the particular condition is a threat to life.

Inmates have certain specific rights in this area. For example, they must be informed of reasons for medical examinations. Sometimes, the exams are required for purposes of classification, or for matters of parole or prison discipline. And they have to give their consent before any testing is done. There are no secrets, either. Any inmate, on written request, may have a copy of all documents referring to both his medical and psychiatric conditions.

There are many sad people in prison, some through remorse for what they have done, others because they view the future as a panorama of hopelessness. Crime in itself is a concealed activity and the inmate, caught in the rigid prison society, is always cautious to conceal his true self from both staff and inmates.

The inmate naturally becomes heavily weighted with loneliness and anger and sometimes, in a desperate effort to relieve his suffering, will resort to suicide. The inmate society may be aware of a likely suicide attempt but accepts this as a personal decision and doesn't interfere with the inmate contemplating it, nor does it report his intentions to anyone. Interestingly enough, only a very small percentage of those who commit suicide have a mental illness.

I have heard of a good many immediate reasons for suicide in prison such as: rejection by the inmate culture, monetary problems in the case of a prison gambling debt, loss of a loved one, and even a simple uncomplicated desire to die. In view of the fact that inmates are utterly alone in their cells for at least twelve hours a day, and that a high percentage of them suffer from fear, anger and loneliness anyway, it is perhaps surprising that there are not more suicides.

Prisoners have little access to drugs and other poisonous substances, have no guns and usually must resort to their own ingenuity to kill themselves. Strangulation is the number one cause of death in suicides. (Drug overdoses and self-inflicted wounds come next.) The only requirement for success is privacy. Any type of rope, wire, tie, bed sheet, shoelace, or belt may be used. And all of them have been used.

Careful planning assures a successful suicide. Inmates will tell you the conventional method is to attach a rope securely to an overhead pipe, get up on a chair, tie the rope around your neck with a firm knot and then kick away the supporting chair. It takes a minimum of five minutes to assure death.

Prison suicides usually cause little or no disturbance among the general inmate population. They will only reveal knowledge of an impending suicide if the person contemplating the act is a *bug*, or otherwise of unsound mind. In such cases inmates may attempt to alert the authorities. If the potential suicide appears to know what he's doing, he'll be left to his own devices, as it were.

It's interesting to note that the day after a suicide is just another day. It's business as usual throughout the institution. News of an inmate's suicide creates as much stir as a battle casualty in war time. Someone may announce, "well, old so-and-so is gone," and the response will be an indifferent shrug and a casual "yeah, poor old Percy. Tough shit."

Life is cheap in a penitentiary, and my files are bulging with evidence attesting to this.

For example, I have this typical report from a Coroner's Jury: "(The inmate), aged forty-nine, died April 6, 1964, from an overdose of carbon tetrachloride (cleaning fluid). Investigation revealed that the inmate, who had worked two years as an office cleaner, had laboriously collected the fluid from bottled supplies in each office of the institution."

It took six ounces of carbon tetrachloride to damage his kidneys beyond repair. Imagine this individual painstakingly collecting his death potion over a period of two years, then killing himself as he planned.

There was Doug, twenty-nine, serving an indefinite sentence as a sex offender. The Coroner's Report said that he died at 7:24 p.m. November 7, 1974, from a self-inflicted overdose of methyl hydrate (rubbing alcohol), obtained through "devious channels" – from an inmate messenger who distributed cleaning supplies to various areas of the prison.

There is a terseness, a matter-of-factness to these reports: "(The inmate,) 50, in a medium security institution, exhibiting no suicidal tendencies, tied his shoelaces together and, using a four-inch pencil in tourniquet fashion, he died on his own bed during noon rest period."

Some inmates go about the business of suicide quietly, almost with dignity, as the inmate in this last report did. Others end it all angrily, as in the case of an inmate of the Federal Prison for Women.

This forty-one year-old prisoner had a tendency to threaten other inmates, and as a consequence she wound up in dissociation. At 11:30 one night in June 1979 she hanged herself in her cell. She left a note for the guards that read: "I killed myself to get you screws into a shit bucket."

Very few suicides command the nearly-unanimous interest of the prison population.

An unlikely candidate for this distinction was a man whom no one would have figured, at least during his early years, as a potential inmate in a penitentiary. Whatever signs there might have been to indicate future problems obviously went undetected.

Richard was one of two well-to-do sons of a prominent Toronto family. Upper middle class Toronto. Rosedale, or some such place. The brothers were in advertising. They drank their martinis very dry, rim-frosted, a twist, at good places. Everybody in the business knew them.

Then one day, it happened. The bad seed that the criminologists tell you someone should have spotted earlier showed up in Richard. It surfaced when he attempted to rob a corner store in Toronto.

As a result of his brief criminal adventure, Richard, the black sheep of the family, was sentenced to six years in Kingston Penitentiary.

There he gave full rein to his contemptible nature. He was a manipulator and he soon conned my old friend Dr. Maurice O'Connor, K.P.'s pioneer psychiatrist, into devoting a great deal of time to him. He also managed to convince Maurice that he had seen the error of his ways.

As a consequence of his supposed rehabilitation, three years later, with the good wishes of the prison administration, Richard was released on what was then known as a ticket-of-leave, the equivalent of today's parole. Tickets-of-leave were coveted in the early 1960's because they were issued sparingly. Richard received one because both O'Connor and the padre were impressed by his exemplary behavior. Both agreed that Richard was the type of inmate who warranted a "break."

Well, Richard said goodbye to his friends at K.P., took off for Toronto and almost immediately became involved in another robbery. Within a matter of days he was back at Kingston Penitentiary, as a rather sheepish returnee, I might add, since he had betrayed the trust of the psychiatrist and the padre, and had, by reneging on the terms of his ticket-of-leave, made it more difficult for other inmates to obtain the privilege. Richard had now incurred the wrath of the police, the prison authorities, the psychiatrist - and the inmates themselves.

Another three years passed. Richard, now a low-profile prison personality, was assigned to a penitentiary work force whose job it was to pick apples on a farm at Smithfield, some eighty miles away. Richard and his buddies picked fruit for a week. Then, one Tuesday, he complained of headache and nausea, and asked an officer to drive him to a nearby house, where he could get a drink of water. The officer agreed, but on the way Richard pulled a knife on him and ordered the officer to drive him to Toronto. There, Richard abandoned the truck and attempted yet another robbery. He was apprehended and once again returned to K.P.

Richard's escapade had now involved him in hostage-taking; it had also ruined the whole apple-picking venture for the other inmates, and they all returned to the prison with loss of this farm work privilege.

Inmates don't like to be played for suckers by one of their own, so Richard was placed on the black list, then put in protective custody because he was so universally hated. Because the inmates had *dummied up* on him, Richard became so depressed that he had to be moved to the psychiatric ward.

On the night of August 27, 1961, Henderson, the hospital officer, discovered Richard in an apparent semi-bewildered state and began to check on him at forty-five-minute intervals. During one of these intervals, Richard fashioned a rope; one end he tied around his neck, the other to a radiator pipe. By constantly turning his entire body over and over and over, Richard managed to hang himself - his head two inches from the ground.

The Coroner arrived some time later and the attendants placed Richard's body on a stretcher. I have many strange memories of life in prison, but none stranger, I think, than the spectacle of the Coroner's attendants carrying Richard's body past the cells of the prisoners who had come to hate him.

As Richard made his last escape from K.P. the inmates began a dirge that sent a shudder through me. In unison, their voices grave and muted, they sang a parody of the old 'Tom Dooley' song..."Hang down your head, hang down your head in shame."

* * *

Self-mutilation is always a problem among prison inmates, although it is rare in private practice. In the outside world, the gesture of cutting one's wrists is a dramatic announcement of one's desperate unhappiness. In my own private practice, I have seen only one case of slashing, committed by a very angry thirty-year-old woman.

In prison the threat to self-mutilate is always clear, with a specific element of manipulation involved. The individual is stating what he wants and spelling out what he will do if he doesn't get it. There is a distinct, dangerous and threatening manner evident in his activities.

Slashing involves about one per cent of the prison population, and it does nothing to enhance an inmate's status. Usually a razor blade is used to cut the inner forearm; occasionally the chest is slashed. Incisions can measure six to ten inches, and often tendons, arteries and nerves are severed. Interestingly, legs are not usually injured.

An inmate who resorts to slashing may describe feelings of anger and pain throughout his body, sensations that become so unbearable that he may hit the walls with his fists or smash his head against a door, prior to the actual slashing. By inflicting outward pain on himself he is attempting to relieve the indescribable inner pain that torments him.

There is no clinical explanation for slashing.

"I feel so pent up," said one man, "that I have to slash myself to get relief."

Another individual offered this almost melodramatic diagnosis. "It's almost as if I were declaring myself the enemy, whom I must attack for causing me so much trouble. I don't try to kill myself. But I feel so awful that I have to inflict real pain to get a sort of release from the terrible sensations."

Psychiatrically, slashing is not a mental illness per se, but individuals who resort to such self-injury always have a history of rebellious, destructive behavior in childhood and violent temper tantrums in adolescence. Slashing is simply another manifestation of anti-social behavior.

Swallowing foreign objects is another manipulative action carried out by that one per cent of the inmates whose quiet manner often hides a terrible anger. A swallower "does his trick" then reports the act to someone in authority, and a series of X-ray studies follow the progress of spoons, knives, forks, bolts, needles, pieces of wire or razor blades through his system.

These inmates never regard themselves as suicidal, and actually become extremely alarmed if they feel that they're in any danger of dying. Their actions are cries for attention, and manipulative in that swallowers usually are hospitalized and undergo surgery, obliterating their prison tensions for a time.

The champion swallower of all time has to be Morris, a twenty-eight-year-old inmate serving a twenty-year sentence for murder with another murder charge in the United States facing him upon his release.

Morris swallowed foreign objects so often that eventually the surgeons notified him - by formal letter no less - that his abdominal wall was such a mass of scar tissue that no healthy skin could be found for further surgery. Morris finally decided to abandon the operating room in favor of the dull routine of general prison life.

In my private practice, one of my patients, a severely depressed sixty-year-old woman, broke her water glass, wrapped the fragments in wet toilet tissue and swallowed them. She died six days later of multiple perforations of the bowel.

Strangely enough, no inmate has ever swallowed glass fragments or anything else that can't be viewed on X-ray.

We can't discuss the prison mind without examining briefly what is perhaps the greatest of all dreams of the incarcerated - escape. For most inmates it is just that - an impossible dream. A fantasy to while away the endless, monotonous hours of captivity. Everyone wants out, but not everyone attempts an escape.

As we've seen, there is more than one mode of "escape." Death by suicide is the "great escape." And for some inmates this is a bigger production than simply slashing or hanging or drinking cleaning fluid.

Jacques, twenty-two, who was serving a life sentence for the murder of a woman, became involved in a hostage-taking while in prison and eventually wound up at Millhaven Institution. Psychiatrically, he exhibited no particular mental aberrations, although his "fixed from under" stare produced a feeling of disquiet in others.

It was Jacques' deep-rooted conviction, however, that he needed psychiatric treatment, despite the absence of disease symptoms. He was therefore sent to the Mental Health Center at Penetang. Two months later he was back, labelled "non-psychotic and not treatable."

Next, he demanded a transfer to the Regional Psychiatric Centre. Once again I made the necessary arrangements, on the remote chance that he might be paranoid, despite previous diagnoses to the contrary. Not long after he was back complaining that the centre couldn't give him the treatment that he knew he needed.

During my bi-monthly sessions with Jacques I was never sure that I would survive his frustrations. Sometimes psychiatrists, despite their objectivity, become more deeply involved with their patients than they intend. Perhaps that was why Jacques, during a rather heavy session, decided to confide in me.

He had thought it all out very carefully; he was going to get himself killed while attempting to escape. Specifically, his intention was that he'd get shot while scaling the inner barrier. Obviously, he saw death as his final escape. But also, he no doubt felt that his death would spark some sort of investigation, and it would come out that he had been denied the psychiatric treatment he believed he needed.

In true fink fashion I reported his plan to the warden.

A couple of days later, at two in the afternoon, my patient went over the inner twelve-foot chain link fence. As he mounted the second fence, the tower guard fired a shot into the ground. Almost paralyzed with fear, Jacques simply fell off the fence, fractured his ankle, and was helped to the infirmary by the officers he had thought would shoot him.

During the next six weeks he became morose and irritable; on the occasion that I saw him after his abortive escape attempt he asked to be transferred to British Columbia, where he felt he would receive proper psychiatric care.

When no transfer was forthcoming, his behavior became more aggressive, particularly toward the other prisoners, and this precipitated a near-fatal attack by an unnamed inmate. He was stabbed repeatedly in the arms, chest and abdomen, and was saved from death only by the quick action and skill of the correctional officers who carried him to the medical centre. He was moribund upon arrival there but was skillfully resuscitated. Upon recovery he was given a transfer – but it wasn't the transfer he had wanted. Instead of sending him to British Columbia, authorities moved him to Québec.

Technically, Jacques was sane, but I'm convinced that deep down he was a demented, tortured man.

A killing in the penitentiary creates as much stir as does a suicide. It's just another incident, and not even thought of in terms of "murder". Inmates, if they speak of him at all, refer to a murder victim as having been *topped*, *knocked off* or *dumped*.

Suspected killers are seldom successfully prosecuted. No inmate will volunteer any information regarding a killing; to expose a killer would be courting sudden death. The inmates have their own version of the three monkeys: "didn't see nothing, didn't hear nothing, won't say nothing."

The exception to this is the case of a vicious unprovoked attack without any cause. In such a situation, an inmate may decide to give evidence in court, feeling the attack was unjustified.

Institutional killings are swift and merciless, and seldom is the victim surprised. More than once I have knelt beside the still-warm body of an inmate, blood oozing from a knife wound in his chest, and pronounced him dead. Moments before, twenty-eight inmates, released from their cells, were on their way to a work assignment. In this brief interval of movement the assassin swiftly dispatched his victim, mingled once more with the shuffling inmates, and went on to his assignment. Such is inmate justice.

There are few random, motiveless killings in prison. A crime may appear casual but there is almost always a reason behind the act.

Every new arrival - particularly a transferee from a maximum security institution - is potential trouble. He may have a personal grudge against an established inmate, or he may have taken on a contract to "settle accounts" on behalf of an inmate in another prison.

"Confrontation killings" are almost commonplace and may result from even a minor disagreement. Such killings are done without stealth; some are almost gladiator-like.

The killing of a new inmate who has committed an "unacceptable" crime is looked upon as an execution. The victim may be a well-publicized sex-offender whose crime is regarded by the other inmates as totally abhorrent.

Some twelve years ago, an accountant who had taken Boy Scouts on weekend camping trips and then molested them, arrived at Kingston Penitentiary to serve a ten-year sentence. His sentence was terminated after forty-eight days inside.

* * *

If suicides and slashings are accepted as part of the prison culture by the inmates, they are likely to be considered less casually in the press. With predictable regularity editorial writers declare that something - no one's ever sure what - must be done to right the wrongs behind our prison walls.

When well-meaning members of coroners' juries suggest that a particular suicide victim should have been in a mental institution rather than a prison, I sympathize with their indignation. And I concede that a closer watch must be kept on certain inmates, and that surely many prison tragedies could be averted.

But what could we have done to prevent the suicide death of Sammy in Joyceville Institution in 1979?

I'll let John McKenna, then assistant Crown Attorney for Frontenac County (the Kingston area) answer that question, as he did in the Whig-Standard, November 8, 1979:

"I have been involved in a number of inquests into prison suicides and have been forced to conclude reluctantly that if someone is intent on committing suicide, there is very little that can be done to prevent it.

"It would be necessary to post a guard beside the prisoner for every second of every day. If the prisoner were not serious about suicide before this procedure, I suggest to you that after a week of this twenty-four-hour-a-day scrutiny of his every movement he would cry 'cruel and unusual punishment' and probably welcome the idea of death.

"I've discovered, from past experience, that removing all horizontal bars in a cell will not prevent a determined man from committing suicide. I recently attended a Coroner's Inquest where it was established that an inmate (Sammy) had hanged himself by the simple expedient of tieing one end of his shoelace around a vertical pipe and the other end tightly around his neck.

"He passed out in a matter of seconds, and the shoelace tightened about his neck. He had hanged - his head only six inches from the floor.

"One can only conclude, then, that security and cell structure are important, but obviously no solution. The tormented life of (the inmate) most certainly could not have been saved by such superficial expedients. To decide whether or not this young man's death might have been prevented, we must consider his life."

What did drive Sammy to take his own life at the ripe old age of twenty-one?

The hard-liners will tell you that no one forced Sammy to join the Joyceville fraternity. And who can argue with that? Of course no one coerced Sammy into the institution. Sammy was a thief, for which offence he was serving time in prison. Pure and simple. But is it really that simple?

We can only guess at what secret torments raged within Sammy, but we do know the salient facts of his life. We know that he entered the institution when he was hardly more than a boy, to serve five years for robbery. We know that he suffered great embarrassment from a severe case of acne, and that he was partially alienated from his family.

We also know that on several occasions Sammy was savagely beaten and raped - the fate of so many young men who end up in prison.

Had he been outside prison walls, Sammy would doubtless have taken up with a girl he'd have called his "old lady." But inside, he had a male friend he called his "old man". In a typical penitentiary arrangement, Sammy's "old man" (he actually was an older man) offered his young friend protection from the prison toughs in return for sexual favors.

It's a matter of tradition that women are segregated from men in the prison system - from the local pokey to the maximum security penitentiary. Unfortunately, we don't segregate the young, virile new inmates from the prison-wise older men who seek their sexual favors.

Sammy continued his relationship with his "old man" until the latter was transferred to Millhaven, at which time Sammy became despondent, dependent on sleeping pills and tranquilizers, and was placed in segregation to protect him from the other inmates.

He had been raped and abused, physically and mentally, and now, in isolation, he was unable to pull himself out of his deep depression. On November 7, 1979, Sammy hanged himself in his cell. Guards found this note:

"Well, it's nearing that time, so goodbye, and one last thing. I don't know where I'm going to be buried, but what I want is for everyone to plan an evening at Grandma and Grandpa's house and I want Grandma to make a meal of her best pancakes in the country and everyone is to make a pig of himself. That's my last request."

There is a footnote to this story. Grandma did make pancakes - stacks of them. And members of the family and friends gathered from all over. Said Grandma of that day, "They sure ate a mess of pancakes. Never before in my whole life did I ever see anyone eat as many of those things as they did."

**CHAPTER 14**

# Special Cases

Russel was one of those inmates we refer to as a "special handling case." It's a term that means exactly what it says and in effect, warns custodial people that they are dealing with someone who requires a full quota of supervision.

Russel was doing eighteen years for bank robbery but that really wasn't the problem. Our institutions are home to a good many bank robbers. They are not a new brand of criminal. The problem was that this individual was confined to Kingston Penitentiary's East Cell Block, the psychiatric wing, as a dangerous inmate.

From time to time, these special handling cases request particular psychiatric help. I had seen Russel on various occasions and listened to a good many of his problems but this day, he was considerably more agitated than usual.

"I've had a lot of rough times, Doc," he said, sinking wearily into the chair across the desk from me, "but this time..." He paused to wet his lips. "This is the first time I've had to lean on someone."

He was tall, thin, fifty-two years of age, with hollow eyes, a hoarse voice and a used-up look about him. He was an intense person, and one to be taken seriously.

"Lean?" I repeated.

"I've got a problem that I can't do anything about and it makes me furious. In fact, I think maybe I'm going nuts."

He was looking for medication to cool him down and I gave him a seven-day prescription. At the end of the week he was back in my office.

"Doc, I'm no better," he said, throwing up his arms. "I'm frustrated, upset." He stopped to find the right words. "Pissed-off. Know what I mean?"

Russel wasn't looking for more medication, as many others do. He wanted to talk. He wanted to tell me what it was that was screwing up his head. It was his armored truck heist near Windsor, the caper that sent him to jail, and it had him pretty worked up.

"It was a $28,000 score," he confided.

He waited to let the words sink in. I finally nodded.

"Well, they never found the loot," he said with a kind of grinning pride. "You know why, Doc?" You know why they never found it?"

I shook my head.

"They never got it because I buried it the next morning. You know where, Doc? Near the Scarborough Golf Club. Then I got on the train and went back to Windsor. I was living in a boarding house there and that afternoon the cops arrived and took the place apart. They also took me apart. They beat three teeth out of the front of my face and caved in my ribs. But, you know what, Doc? I never told them where the money was. I had this idea, see? That dough was going to look after me when the arthritis took over. It was like one of them retirement savings plans."

"Well, a guy's got to look ahead," I said facetiously.

"Hold on, Doc," he said, "that ain't the end of the story. I got a letter from my mother on Monday, and she knows where I stashed the stuff, and Jesus Christ, you wouldn't believe it, the goddam bulldozers are in there levelling the whole area for a supermarket."

He was holding his face in the palms of his hands and shaking his head.

"That great big elm tree. They cut it down. They tore up the ground and now some stupid bugger's going to find my $28,000. All those bucks gone. Nothing left for retirement."

Three days later, I saw him again. The histrionics were over. He was calm and collected, obviously having decided he might as well accept the inevitable. He looked at me for a moment and shrugged his shoulders.

"You know, Doc, I been thinking," he said. "It took me just thirty-five minutes to pull off that job. It's not like I had the money for a long time. And besides, I'm still a long way from retirement."

* * *

When a man starts reciting the story of his life, his friends are likely to regard him as an egotist, or eccentric. If he starts talking about his frustrations, his disappointments, and the sadness of his life, they almost certainly will consider him a bore, or at the very least a pessimist. They might even stifle yawns.

I know that sometimes I surprise some of my acquaintances. I say acquaintances because most of my friends have overcome their tendency to be surprised by me. I guess, of course, that people who hobnob with criminals may be, for want of a better word, "different," even if the hobnobbing is done in a professional capacity.

Crime and criminals, however, fascinate people, with the result that sometimes when I'm entertaining, I get around to talking about, well yes, crime and criminals.

"Hey, Scotty," someone is bound to call out, using my nickname, "tell them about the time you were best man at a murderer's wedding."

I'd rather talk about horses, which I love, but as I say, there is a fascination for crime and I did stand up for such a man once. It was a long time ago – in fact back in the 1950's, soon after I started out at Kingston Penitentiary.

Jerry had killed someone in Toronto, had been sentenced to be hanged and had had his sentence commuted to one of life. Locked up at K.P., he kept thinking about this girl back home. Finally he took his problem up with the prison padre, Rev. John Wylie. He was in love with the girl, he said, and wanted to marry her. The couple had, in fact, planned to get married prior to the trial.

Warden Art Jarvis gave his consent, and one afternoon we all found ourselves in a big room with gray pine flooring above the north gate entrance. Being sentimental about weddings and such things, I had to count it as a special experience. The bride was a pretty girl of about twenty-four who arrived early and sat in a cane chair until her husband-to-be arrived with an escort of officers. She had brought carnation boutonnières and placed one on Jerry 's blue prison shirt and the other on my lapel.

Padre Wylie spoke briefly about the significance of marriage and then performed the ceremony. Later, he produced a small white cake and coffee. The whole ceremony, including the wedding party, had lasted about half an hour. It ended with some stifled tears as guards escorted Jerry back down the winding stairs and to his cell block.

The padre and I walked the new bride through the big gates to the street and said goodbye and good luck. I don't recall any exchange of words between the padre and me afterward, but I do remember the small grin on his face. I think he really enjoyed performing that ceremony.

My friends are constantly surprised at the variety of people I know, but then a great many different personalities have passed through my office over the years and some of them, I have to admit, have been rather strange.

Take Bruce, for instance, the man who kept pretending to hang himself and finally did.

Bruce, raised in Toronto, was seven when he went to his first foster home. He moved from home to home and finally did stretches in training schools and reformatory. He was twenty-eight when I first got to know him and serving a ten-year term for manslaughter. Being in prison didn't bother him. He was a big man – six feet, one inch tall and about 180 pounds – with a strong homosexual drive. His life was an incessant round of partner-hunting but because he had a knuckle-fisted kind of affection, the relationships he established were always short-lived.

Big though he was, there were bigger men at K.P. at the time and occasionally, when his sexual appetite was overly-strong, one of them would tell him to lay off the kids. Every time he was reprimanded this way he would routinely stage a supposed suicide attempt the next evening. The purpose of the act was to gain admittance to the psychiatric wing, from where he could probably win a transfer to another range where he wasn't in trouble.

He had been admitted to the psychiatric wing on seven different occasions while he was at K.P. and never would confess that he had staged any of the attempted suicides. But Officer George Gilmour began studying the various incidents and came up with a scenario that was formally accepted by the authorities.

This is how Gilmour put the story together:

Prison routine required that two officers make the rounds of the ranges every twenty minutes at night, as part of the institutional security program. Each range gate was opened by a large key. Opening a range was a noisy affair, alerting the sleepless among the inmates that the guards were making their routine check.

Bruce, of course, was well aware of the routine. He would fashion a noose and hang it from a pipe. Then he would stand on a chair and wait for the sound of the key opening the range. When he heard the sound, he stepped off the chair, dropping his head into the noose. It took about a minute for the officers to reach his cell, see him hanging there and cut him down. His removal to hospital for observation then was assured.

It was a perfect plan. It worked every time. Then, on the night of June 9, 1969, something went wrong.

Bruce set up his noose and stood on the chair. A few minutes later he heard the great key turning the lock to open the range. He stepped off the chair and slipped his head into the noose.

As the officers entered the range they spotted a man in one of the first cells in the midst of an epileptic seizure. They opened his cell door and remained with him until he had recovered. Then they proceeded with their check of the rest of the range.

When they got to Bruce's cell, they found him dangling in the noose - by now a familiar sight. They cut him down but this time it was too late. He had been hanging there for several minutes and he was dead.

The story of Bruce is the only case in my bulging files where suicide was not suicide but just a matter of bad timing. A coroner's inquest ruled it had been a matter of death by misadventure.

* * *

Then there was Tommy, a bright, witty man of thirty-two with a propensity for being mischievous. A manic depressive, he would have one period every year during which he would become withdrawn and depressed. These cycles were regularly attended by criminal acts which were really not dangerous to anyone, but which got him into trouble with the law just the same.

Tommy arrived at K.P. in 1967 on a two-year sentence for threatening a bus driver, and he didn't understand his predicament at all. He told me all he had done was ride a bus with a shotgun across his knees. And what was wrong with that? He went around armed because he didn't like pigeons.

I saw a lot of Tommy and, as I had suspected, there was more than pigeons and riding shotgun involved. An apprentice engraver at a jewelry shop, he had taken all his employer's diamonds out of the safe because "something told me the shop was going to be robbed." Tommy was a pretty fair engraver and, on occasion, turned out some excellent $20 bills. The RCMP were aware of his activities but could never find his plates.

He completed his stint at K.P. without particular incident and was released. Six months later he was back to serve a six-year sentence for hijacking a bus with twenty-four passengers aboard. He explained to his passengers that a rival bus company had planned to burn the vehicle as an act of intimidation and he was trying to save bus and passengers from harm. He was arrested whcn the bus finally ran out of gas.

Back at K.P. he functioned well for two years. Then one day, without any warning, he declared he was God and attempted to amputate his penis. I never did discover why, as God, he felt he had to perform surgery on his genitals. The act assured his hospitalization in the psychiatric unit for another year.

In 1974 he returned home on parole and, within a few days, confessed to his parole officer that he had killed a man some twenty-five years earlier. Again the long arm of the law scooped him up. Tommy was a man with vivid recall and he told police in detail how he had accidentally shot a taxi driver as he stepped out of the cab back in 1950. A coroner's inquest had ruled the death accidental but now, twenty-five years later, he was held for the fall assizes of the Supreme Court of Ontario, charged with murder. It was a complicated case, with judge and jury having to weigh facts already a quarter of a century old. The trial ended in conviction but an appeal resulted in his getting a new trial. This time, the judge decided there was not enough evidence to proceed with the case and it was dismissed.

Tommy was a free man. Well, not quite. He was going through an emotional period (aggravated by his involvement in two new trials) and the Parole Service decided it would be in his best interest to serve out the balance of his parole behind bars. He went to Collins Bay Penitentiary where he served out his time in peace and dignity. In May 1976 he was released to start a new life on the outside.

Tommy got a warm farewell from those of us who had come to know him (and perhaps even to understand him) but he wasn't the least bit happy about leaving. Five days later, at ten o'clock at night, there was a pounding on the door of Collins Bay. Through the bullet-proof glass window the night keeper saw a familiar face.

"Jesus Christ, let me in."

Tommy was waving his arms in the air like a crazy man and the keeper opened the door to him.

"Let me in. The whole goddamn place out there has gone crazy."

The keeper admitted him and I saw him the following day. He had cooled down by then but it was obvious he wasn't ready for the rat race of free society. He needed further psychiatric help. In a way he had come back home, where everybody knew him, and where many liked him.

"Do you know why I wanted back in The Bay, Doc?" he asked me later.

"You tell me," I suggested.

"Well, here," he said seriously, "you can live like a human being."

* * *

Science plays a role in my work and I like to think I can classify most of my patients. I thought, for instance, that I had Reggie pegged and found I was a little off base.

Reggie was twenty and an unusually tall person at six feet seven inches. He had an athletic body but his facial features lacked warmth and expression. He moved slowly in an uncoordinated fashion and his misshapen teeth and unruly hair placed him one focus away from a horror creature.

He had taken two guards as hostages and in May 1980 he was placed in the Special Handling Unit at Millhaven Institution as an exceptionally dangerous, impulsive person. At his own request, I saw him at weekly intervals. Actually, he was of special interest to me because I had studied tall inmates over a ten-year period and had drawn a carefully-detailed chromosomal picture of them.

It seemed to me Reggie was a likely person to have the X YY Syndrome, the extra Y suggesting a possible potential for criminality in the individual.

I reviewed the chromosomal theory with him, describing the physical appearance and various other characteristics of the X YY subject, and he listened intently. They he asked to be allowed to recap the information in his own words. I gave him the go-ahead.

"You say an X YY person is six feet two inches, or more, right?"

"Right."

"You say he's not overly bright?"

"Correct."

"You tell me I've got hypogonads and a small penis?"

I paused, wondering whether I should have gotten into the chromosomal theory with him at all, violent as he was.

"Well, I'm going to tell you something, Doc. My knockers are like golf balls and my penis ain't no hypo. Matter of fact, it's caused quite a commotion in different places. So, I ain't got no X YY disease. Get it, Doc?"

I nodded. "Got it."

* * *

If I sometimes fall down on my chromosomes, I seldom make a mistake where personality is concerned. I knew I was right about Leslie, the police investigation notwithstanding.

Leslie stepped off an eastbound trolley at Coxwell and Danforth in Toronto shortly before Christmas 1967 and was arrested by police who charged him with armed robbery of two drug stores, a supermarket and a small grocery store. Three victims identified him positively in a police lineup and he wound up with a six-year stretch in prison.

He requested to see me because of symptoms of anxiety, tension and sleeplessness. He denied the whole series of robberies and claimed he had been railroaded. He had no criminal record and, in fact, had been a well-paid employee of a Bloor Street business machine company, he said.

After three interviews, I was convinced. This man lacked all of the personality traits of the robber. I was even more convinced when his girl friend agreed to come down to Kingston to talk to me. She reaffirmed my concept of his passive nature.

In brief, Leslie was not a robber.

I then called the robbery division of the Toronto Metropolitan Police and two detectives showed at at K.P. They had full notes on the case, including details of the identification in the lineup, and couldn't see how a mistake could have been made.

I explained my concept. Certain types of people commit certain types of crimes, I pointed out. An armed robber is direct, aggressive and fearless. A fraud offender is passive, effusive, flattering and manipulative. A thief is an uncertain, inadequate person.

Leslie was none of these.

Fortunately, the robberies continued to happen in east-end Toronto and police finally arrested the real robber. He knew Leslie had been jailed wrongly and decided to give the police a full statement of his criminal activities. The police said he looked so much like Leslie that the robbery victims might well be excused for making an error in identification.

Of course, one can be easily confused watching a police lineup. But personalities never lie.

**CHAPTER 15**

# Brew Masters

Henry was known as the Brew Master of Kingston Penitentiary. He was a short-statured man of fifty with a deep voice and a hoodlum smile, and he looked just like a bootlegger should look.

Bootleggers and brew masters are at different ends of the social scale but that was all right with Henry because he was both. Actually, he was what is generally referred to in the joints as a *jail merchant.* He sold his products by the quart and delivered them to his customers in small plastic bags or in long, cigar-like balloons.

Henry did little work in prison but managed to function very well behind the façade of range cleaner and kitchen helper. A thief by outside profession, he was respected and trusted widely by the inmates. However, he was a firm believer in the old saying that credit makes bad friends and insisted on immediate payment upon delivery. It had to be street money and in cash – no promises, no trades, no rebates.

As both brew master and bootlegger, he believed that his customers should get their money's worth. He had two prices: one dollar and two dollars a quart. The price depended on what you ordered. He produced several "brands" of alcohol and each was classed by time of fermentation. Each type was identified as being a five-day green brew, a seven-day brew, or a ten-day ripe brew.

Henry peddled potato peeling brew, breakfast "Cheerios" brew, orange peel brew, prune, peach and other fermentable concoctions. It wasn't exactly like the drinks your favorite bartender would make on the outside but some of it was pretty fair. The potato brew, Henry would tell you, was not entirely unlike vodka in taste. The prune brew had its own special feature – there was no froth on the surface. And Henry would beam with pride when he talked of his Ten Gallon Brew. It contained, among other good things, orange juice fortified with Vitamin C.

His suppliers, by necessity, were also his customers, since he collected his ingredients from other inmates. He paid for the goods he needed by discounting his product to those who supplied him. The discounts were usually modest, Henry believing that since he took most of the risk, he should be entitled to most of the profits.

One day in 1973 Henry showed up in the psychiatric ward as a patient. He was, he said, suffering from anxiety. Well, he was anxious all right but not in the psychiatric sense. He was anxious to open a branch operation for his brewing business. He managed to find just what he wanted – a cell at the end of a range which had a ventilator flue eight by twelve inches, running from the floor to the roof.

Over a period of three months, he played the role of the nervous inmate. "Yeah, Doc, I think I'm a little better," he said in one of our early interviews. Later he would say "You know, Doc, I'm getting better and better every day."

Actually he was getting better and better – at making brew. In his quiet little cell in the psychiatric ward, away from the interruptions of the open population, he was making a gallon every ten days.

He would drain his brew into a tin container with a screw-on top and place it in the ventilator flue. In ten days time, he would push the container up the flue and place a new brew below it. Eventually, he would have eight gallons stored away like this, with the last one firmly wedged above the inlet to the ventilator. In the same flue, he would dig a small recess between the stones, where he could hide his street money.

It all worked well – until one hot afternoon in June.

There was a muffled explosion and a rush of liquid in Henry's cell. The smell of sour green alcohol was nauseating. The guards on the range, who had smelled sour alchohol before, came running.

What had happened was that Henry had been careless. He had screwed one of the can lids on too tightly, thus allowing a build-up of pressure. The result was the explosion and deluge. The wet brew loosened the wedge below the latest batch and, to the brew master's horror, everything came sliding down the ventilator, including some thirty sticky one-dollar bills.

Henry, always one to take adversity with a smile, quipped, "The revenuers aren't going to like this one."

The authorities laid disciplinary charges against him and then transferred him to Joyceville Institution, which has a large farm annex and provides food for a great many prisoners. Henry was just short of ecstatic with the transfer.

"Vegetables, cereals, fruits," he exclaimed in obvious delight when I met him again later. "They got everything at Joyceville."

The problems of brewing in prison are extremely complex. In fact, the brewer has the entire prison staff on his tail all the time. It may be difficult enough collecting the ingredients for a brew – but concealing them is even more difficult. One inmate I knew liked "Cheerios" brew and kept his cereal (which he got for breakfast) in a plastic bag in his pillow. Eventually, he had half a bushel stashed away in his cell. An unexpected cell search found his supplies and he was charged with possession of contraband.

Yeast is one of the important ingredients and its supplies have to be guarded carefully. An inmate of the Prison for Women, who came to me for psychiatric counsel one day, went to great lengths to guard her yeast.

My nostrils kept twitching during the interview and at one point I said, "I smell something a little musty, no offence to you."

"You're right, Doc," she smiled, unbuttoning her blouse and drawing a small plastic bag from out of the fold of her bosom. "Nobody's gonna get their hands on my yeast. I'm riggin' up a brew for the weekend."

Most of the brews are planned in terms of weekend drinking. Everyone in prison knows this and the authorities would put an end to the practice if they could. But the problem is that if they do manage to find a batch fermenting and confiscate it, there is sure to be another, and another and another in the works somewhere else. Inmates, for the most part, are conscious of the problems of institutional drinking and abide by one major unwritten rule: drink in moderation. There is very rarely a case of drunkenness in prison.

Henry has passed out of the prison system and I have no idea where he is, but before leaving he dropped into my office with recipes for two of his favorite concoctions: his famous Prune Brew and Ten Gallon Brew. The following are his very own instructions:

**Prune Brew**

1. Boil prunes, strain off juice.
2. To pulp, add: Water – 1 gallon
   Yeast – medium amount
   Sugar – two cups
   Orange or grapefruit juice
   3 cans (medium)
3. Let set for eight to twelve days

**Ten Gallon Brew**

1. Orange juice fortified with Vitamin C - 6 small cans
2. Yeast pellets, or real yeast, or soft centre from loaf of bread
3. Sugar – 2 cups per gallon – 20 cups
4. Put in warm place for four days.

Henry may have been one of the great prison brewers of them all, but life doesn't stand still and new brewers mature. Today, every institution has its own Brew Master and each is proud of his work. There is a new sophistication, too, in the use of names for the brews and in ingredients used. The following recipes are rated A-1 by inmates:

**Ketchup Chateau.**

Time to mature: 3-4 days

1. 60 ketchup envelopes (like the kind found in restaurants)
2. A little less than 4 gallons of lukewarm water
3. 6 cups of sugar
4. Fill 4-gallon pail with lukewarm water if no yeast pellets.

Take 6 mashed soft-boiled potatoes. Let set for 48 hours in warm room.
If starter is needed, large jar (2-3 cups) of any kind of fruit and let set for 48 hours before Ketchup Chateau is started.
Strain, throw away solids, and let settle. Ready for use.
Notes: if you leave brew too long, it becomes vinegar.
If brew stops bubbling, stop it and strain.
Don't move it because this will stop the brewing.
If needed to drink, add ice to stop the cooking.
Drink:
Need about 3 cups to feel it.
Large Tom Collins glass of brew is equivalent to a 2 1/2 ounce drink in a tall glass

**Cherry Brandy**

The best and strongest brew
Time to mature: 3 weeks

1. 1 pail of cherries; macerate to pulp
2. Place in plastic 8 gallon milk bag
3. Add 4 gallons of water
4. Add 12 cups of sugar
5. Place in warm area
6. Brew for 21 days.

**Pure Alcohol Brew**

Time to produce: 1-2 days
Cherries, mashed in small amount of fluid
Equipment: Electric kettle
Put brew in kettle. Block off spout. Put tube through spout and let it condense in a cold glass. This is alcohol.
In another version of the same recipe, it is recommended that the brewer stir with one cup of water.

**Potato Brew**

Time to produce: 2 days

1. 14 boiled potatoes, mashed
2. Add yeast if available
3. Add 4 gallons of warm water
4. If starter needed, use 3 shredded wheat cakes

5. Mix up with or without starter
6. Brew for two days, then strain and serve.

* * *

Alcohol is not a real threat to prison life. Like society itself, the prison contains all elements of human expression. One man may sleep with alcohol, a second may become contemplative and a third may become aggressive. In prison, behavioural qualities, not alcohol qualities, form the base line. In prison, alcohol becomes a dangerous weapon when it excites man's mind to hostility, rebellion and defiance; and it can remain undiscovered as long as its worshippers are controlled and reverent.

It's the fermentation process that has obvious complications. The smell of warm yeast, the dullness of carbon gas, and the symbiotic relationship of the peachfly to fermenting fruits, may give the tell-tale clues to the existence of brew alcohol. One observant penal officer determines alcohol on his range by simply watching the peachfly population.

**CHAPTER 16**

# Drugs: Highs and Lows Behind the Walls

Drugs, like alcohol, are used in prison in much the same way as they are in the street, except that there is more sophistication in obtaining, selling and using them. A prisoner lives in a very rigid and uncompromising reality. It is little wonder, then, that he turns to his own devices to search out immediate and available methods which will allow him to escape from his world for a few short hours.

He has a number of channels open to him. The first is to seek out the medical officer who assesses his emotional state and prescribes some relieving medication. Many inmates have ongoing anxiety with accompanying symptoms of headache, restlessness, sleeplessness and irritability. Institutional tensions aggravate these anxieties. To complicate the medical problem, an inmate may have had an extensive experience with alcohol and drugs on the street. His tolerance to stress is thus greatly reduced and he makes frequent demands for medication.

The psychiatrist sees the more resistant cases. From time to time, chronically drug dependent inmates have to be continued on some prescription plan until they have settled into the institution. Some of the more manipulative inmates appear on sick parade with a recitation of symptoms but really are attempting to obtain tranquilizers to use in the barter system of the prison.

These inmates keep their supplies of tranquilizers and sedatives in ample stock. Frequent cell searches find many types of pills hidden away. It must be remembered, of course, that pills are currency. The problem of pill-hoarding has been reduced in the last ten years by placing all drugs in a water solution with the dosage swallowed in front of the medical attendant. But drugs still turn up in cells and along the ranges.

Occasionally, a drug package is thrown over the fence of a prison, or concealed in an incoming vehicle, to be retrieved at some prearranged point. The smuggled sedatives are sold to inmate buyers, and usually saved for weekend consumption. The arrival of new drugs is soon discovered. There are semistuporous inmates, aggressive acts and noisy, profane language.

Drugs are used in general medicine in a wide range of conditions, with secondary and toxic effects carefully assessed. Drugs in the prison world are used in a different way, with the secondary effect often being the object of desire.

An epidemic of hemorrhoids was observed in one institution not so long ago. The condition was treated with hot baths, suppositories with "Gall et Opii" ointment. The medical officer investigated the suspicious circumstances and found the inmates were using the "Gall et Opii" treatment on bread to obtain an opium lift.

Several factors operate in prison pharmacology, which make the use of drugs an enigmatic, paradoxical and controversial problem.

Drugs which have reality-changing effects or comparable toxic effects are always in demand as the dependent inmate seeks release from his anxieties. His frequent appearance on sick parade may be justified, but he is actually trying to find a chemical solution to his problems.

Inmates, not actually ill, may develop artificial complaints to obtain drugs which they can use as currency in the prison barter system. They also may pass their drugs to friends whose "needs" are greater than theirs. Inmates too, may magnify their complaints with a view to "hoarding" their medications against some future date when they may be in short supply, or when problems such as parole turndown, may make reality unacceptable.

Prisoners may use the sick parade as a social forum wherein communication is established with other segregated inmates. Complaints have to be presented to justify their presence. The complaint and the prescriptions are of secondary importance. At times, large sick parades are developed to irritate the medical officer because of some misunderstanding. The officer becomes skilled in this double dealing and never loses the respect of the inmate if he sees through their manipulations.

Sick parades, with demand for drugs, enlarge in numbers when a new or substitute medical officer appears. The inmate population knows it can take advantage of the medical officer who has prescribed only for a general practice.

An inmate may seek his drug choice with the argument that his "doctor in the street" prescribed it, or another prison doctor ordered it for him. There are many requests for amphetamines for narcolepsy, barbituates for some ill-defined epilepsy, and the "maintenance tranquilizer" used in another institution, either penal or mental.

The rapidly reacting pentobarbitals (Seconals, Tuinals) together with the slower acting Amytals are requests of choice. Inmates desire a few moments of relaxation and will fight the soporific effects to enhance their mental ecstasy. These drugs have a high barter value and may even be used intravenously by the resourceful inmate.

Intravenous pentothal gives a prolonged period of relaxation and relief. The motivation for a psychiatric catharsis has not infrequently sprung from the desire for a post-treatment jag.

Tranquilizers have lesser addictive propensities but may form a habit relationship if given over a long period of time. Such tranquilizers as the phenothiazines, and fluphenazines have no exotic effects but, in many instances, place the inmate in a distant and removed state of indifference.

The meprobamates have potentially addicting properties in dependent and alcoholic addicts. The non-barbituate sedative has a useful role but has many inherent problems. A non-controlled drug can be as dangerous as a controlled narcotic if used indiscreetly and routinely.

Such medications include chloral hydrate, methylprylon (Noludar), glutethimide (Doriden), and other similar drugs. These are now recorded in the drug schedule and can be dispensed only with a doctor's signature.

Drug demands may be quite legitimate in obvious situations of emotional stress. The inmate may be shaken up because of disturbing home news, prison difficulties, pre-release jitters, induction tensions. Then there are inmates with prime neurotic histories indicating the need for drug assistance. There may be some dependent,inadequate individuals who can only maintain their health in society, and in prison, through the use of appropriate tranquilizers and sedative drugs.

Similarly, the symptoms of sleeplessness, irritability and complaints of indigestion and tension, need to be checked out for authenticity with appropriate prescription of medication. Medication is never prescribed for prolonged periods of time. Two weeks is a sufficient period, with at least a two-week break before further medication.

The use of cerebral stimulants, the benzedrines, dexedrines and methedrines, have been removed from the drug pharmacopia. The drugs may produce a prolonged period of unreality, during which time the inmate may experience promiscuous, aggressive or violent behavior. The mood elevators cannot be assessed too clearly. The prison world is by nature, depressing. These drugs may temporarily medicate the inmate over a stress period but, in general, are not particularly effective. "Weight losing" drugs must be dispensed with care as the secondary gain from psychic release may be the real goal. In general, the overweight patient should be left to his own resources if he wishes to reduce his weight. Actually, inmates who are overweight are really only marginally so, if they have been in prison for some time, because their access to food is regulated.

In women's institutions, the drug situation is immeasurably complicated by the type of inmate incarcerated. In my experience, the woman offender is a creature of hate, rebellion, conflict and selfishness. Her early history has trained her to resent control and authority. Her feelings of hate are usually so overpowering that she will try any method to relieve her chronic anger. If she has an addiction problem, imprisonment magnifies her tensions, aggravates her pathology and pushes her frantically to chemical adaptation.

The female inmate has no respect for sister inmates, none for the custodial staff and uses the medical department in a demanding and disrespectful manner. She has no understanding of medical ethics, demands attention at all times and insists upon medication as a right totally unrelated to therapeutic principles. She will direct her drives at the nurses and doctors, with ongoing demands for drugs of her choice. If legitimate supplies are not available, other inmates are made to come and ask for medication.

Inmates on day parole are forced to bring drugs into prison. More aggressive inmates may threaten to break up their cells or to slash themselves if drugs are not prescribed. Frequent slashings occur with a view of receiving tranquilizers and sedative drugs as a consequence of their acts.

The female offender feels that drugs are her right, and in consequence, has no judgment or understanding of the dynamics of the medical department. She can never be satisfied in her search for chemical adaptation. Her demands are continuous and unfortunately all too often successful.

A one-month cut-off period every three months is a controlling device to reduce illicit supplies in the population, to remove pressure from the medical staff and, in a devious way, to inform the inmate that she cannot continuously satisfy her demands for chemical adaptation. (The male inmate with his psychological stability and his acceptance of his situation does not present the complex problems of the female prisoner).

Chemicals and chemistry, their combinations and effects, are not known by the average inmate. He hears anecdotes, listens to stories and often, in his desperate loneliness, searches and finds a chemical to solve his temporary anxiety.

Chemicals closely associated with the alcohol formula, the methyl alcohols, paraldehydes, formaldehydes and other aldehyde compounds, together with solutions which have an alcohol evaporative quotient, are soon found to have an inhalant or ingestive quality. The effects of inhalant ether, or ingestive chloral hydrate are soon determined. The inhalation of gasoline fumes from the garage or acetone from the paint shop, and of airplane glue from the wood shop, are all possibilities for the "trip-hungry" inmate. He may ingest liquids which smell like alcohol. Typewriter cleaner fluid with its odd and deadly chemical effects may cause death through liver poisoning. Any chemical, unsupervised in the prison setting, may, in a frantic moment, be used by the inmate in his blind, impulsive and unreasoning search for relief.

These notes are from my files:

**Methyl Alcohol Blindness - Rubbing Alcohol**

Inmate Burt, age thirty-one, drank four ounces of methyl alcohol while employed in the paint shop. In twelve hours he was found with muscle spasm, painful, blurred vision, and vomiting. Stated someone mixed "it" for him and he drank it. Completely blind in two weeks. Background revealed male of limited intelligence and Grade 5 education. He had a long history of intoxication, shopbreaking, robbery, assault and theft. He had no motivation other than "to be a thief." Board of Enquiry noted "drinking people should not be put in jobs where chemicals exist."

**Ethyl Glycol Poisoning - Antifreeze**

A yellowish-green antifreeze obtained from radiator of portable air compressor. Eight inmates drank this fluid. Two drank amounts in excess of six ounces. Within twelve hours both were complaining of abdominal discomfort but seemed in no serious distress. Both died suddenly ten days later. The spree occurred without planning when one inmate saw "antifreeze" marked on a ticket on the radiator cap. Symptoms of vomiting, weakness, fast pulse, rapid respiration, headache and blurred vision were marked. Death occured through severe kidney damage with anuria, with rapidly developing mental condition and coma on the twelfth day. Pharmacology: ethylene glycol is broken down in body to produce oxalic acid. This acid destroys the tubules of the kidney and sets off a general body deterioration with uremia, hepatomegaly, necrosis of the liver, ascites and toxic degeneration of the basal ganglia of the brain.

**Carbon Tetrachloride Poisoning - Cleaning Fluid**

Inmate Barny, a thirty-five year-old inmate was admitted to the prison hospital with marked anxiety and apprehension. He had attended sick parade frequently for the preceding two weeks with symptoms of indigestion and abdominal discomfort. He consumed large quantities of milk. He vomited frequently and, in the next twenty-four hours, became irrational and uncontrollable. Transferred to psychiatric unit with increase in restlessness, irrationality, mental confusion. He was found dead in his hospital cot, on morning rounds, three days later. Cause of death was uncertain at that time. Investigation revealed pneumonia but there was evidence of a blue fluid being ingested. This fluid was later traced to typewriter cleaner fluid with a tetrachloride base. Post mortem revealed acute irritation of the small intestine. Previous history revealed he was of superior intelligence with Grade ten education. Criminal record was extensive; was serving a robbery charge of seven years; had frequent imprisonments.

Carbon tetrachloride is a colorless liquid with a sweet aromatic odour like chloroform, and is used as a solvent for oil, grease etc.. It produces symptoms of headache, nausea, muscle cramps, sleepiness, with uremia, hepatitis and cerebral edema. Death may occur from two to ten days after ingestions.

**Shellac Intoxication (Methyl alcohol solvent)**

A fifty-seven year-old recidivist serving his twenty-third year in prison with some forty offences, had a long history of alcoholism. Background revealed an unsettled home life with Grade seven education. He was unmarried and his employment skills showed no motivation to improve. His whole life centered around an existence with alcohol. In prison, he used shellac as an intoxicating agent. Yellow shellac was mixed with water and stirred to remove the rosin portions. The remainder was strained through bread leaving an alcohol-type solution. A good "jag" was produced. White shellac he stated, couldn't be strained through bread, was very dangerous and made one deathly sick.

**Mice Pellets**

Possessing a strychnine content, these can produce periods of mental excitement. Mild, convulsive reactions occur in the course of their ingestion. In large doses, severe and fatal convulsions occur.

**Mace**

Mace is the aromatic spice of the nutmeg bark and nutmeg seed. A yellowish volatile oil myristic, it produces, in one to six hours, excitement, delirium and unconsciousness. Hepatic necrosis may be fatal. Taken in a small dose in powdered form, it produces a sensation of mental confusion and excitement, not unlike marijuana intoxication.

**Women's Cosmetics**

These usually contain some methyl alcohol-type base. Stick cologne and stick deodorant may be melted down and taken orally. It has a disagreeable taste, is very toxic and results in visual blurring for a number of hours.

**Liquid Perfume**

This is mixed directly with some carbonated drink to produce a relatively short period of euphoria.

**Hair Spray**

With its basic chemical characteristics, it produces a very dangerous and toxic effect. The liquid spray is mixed with hot water. It is very irritating to the throat, produces a period of mental confusion and indifference, with dizziness and blurring of vision. Residual toxic effects have been observed two weeks after ingestion with symptoms of cerebral irritability, increased sensitivity to noise and visual complaints.

**Nail Polish Remover**

With its acetone base, it can be used as an inhalant and has narcotic properties. If inhaled, it produces headaches and dizziness. If ingested, it produces drowsiness and confusion.

**Turpentine**

It can't be considered palatable, but it is used by the inmate by injecting quantities of the liquid into the muscles of the leg. A period of mental confusion and disorientation occurs. Usually the injected area sloughs out in a most painful manner in the subsequent two to three weeks.

Industrial chemicals are extremely dangerous in the prison environment although they may be absolutely necessary in the function of the institution. Any liquid or solid chemical which has any of the characteristics of alcohol may be used to release reality. The inmate knows not, cares not, but searches for his moment of adventure.

**CHAPTER 17**

# The Prison for Women

No matter how often I approach the Federal Prison for Women, each time I experience a strange sense of awe. I've entered that stately structure at all times of the year, but sometimes, in the spring, there is an almost ethereal quality about the massive stone building. Seen in the early morning, as the warm air rolls over the frozen ground, the prison appears to perch on a cloud of fog, suspended above the world.

Built in 1930, and situated a stone's throw from Kingston Penitentiary, the Prison for Women is a sophisticated assembly of stone, thick bars and heavy locks.

The cells are in ranges of twenty, two to each of three floors, thus accommodating one hundred and twenty inmates. A smaller, reinforced section on two levels segregates the trouble-makers – dangerous and intractable women – from the rest of the prisoners. A wooden addition, with larger rooms and windows, can house twenty inmates in modest comfort.

Each cell in the main structure reflects the tastes and personality of its occupant. Drapes behind the bars provide a certain privacy, while personal photographs, magazine clippings, souvenirs and books clutter the cubicles.

In addition to the usual mess halls, workshops and laundries, there is a well-equipped gymnasium for the athletically-inclined, and smaller, adjoining rooms for general recreation, TV viewing and lecture programs. And there's a library that offers the inmates a wide variety of fiction and non-fiction, current magazines and newspapers.

The staff to inmate ratio is two to one, slightly higher than in the institutions for men.

This is the limited world of between eighty and one hundred and forty female inmates (the number varies from month to month, year to year) whose offences range all the way from prostitution and shoplifting to drug trafficking and murder.

I believe every woman in prison represents a protest against the physical and emotional dominance of man. The fleeting charms of woman's physical being exist for a brief stage entrance, while the emotional strife, fears and hurts, which have begun early in childhood, last for a lifetime. Many child-women, or adolescent women are manipulated, used, beaten, controlled and sexually assaulted at the selfish whims of dominant males.

As womanhood arrives, the embitterment and hate is turned back onto the male who is at most a poor adversary to the avenging, criminal woman. Man is a hated object. A woman in a man's world steals from man's business empires. Some forty per cent of women in prison are sentenced for theft, forgery and robbery. Others use men's sexual appetites to advantage in the lucrative call girl and prostitution empires.

An equal percentage of female drug addicts become criminals as they become involved in the illicit drug trade. Twenty per cent of female inmates have convictions for manslaughter and murder and guess who the victims are – males. It must be remembered, however, that women usually murder in a defensive act to protect themselves from physical hurt.

I have seen a large number of female heroin addicts at the Prison for Women who are there because of some offence against the Narcotics Act. Most of the women have been completely exploited by the male sex by the age of ten years. They have learned to survive on the streets, have little schooling, uniformly have left home by the age of twelve and have become professional thieves by fourteen. In the course of events, they add streetwalking and prostitution to their cadre training.

Eventually they are introduced to heroin and find it is the magic needle that removes their hate by producing normal feelings for a few fleeting hours. But soon they are again possessed by hate and again they turn to heroin to relieve it.

They accept their rejection of the males and accept the friendship of their sister addicts. They become a group bonded together by a degree of caring and a warmth and need for each other.

All my heroin-addicted patients have tense, defensive personalities, and are thin and gaunt in appearance. They befriend each other and usually find a mate to support their insecurity. Many return to the street as a couple.

I call them the 4-H Girls. Hate, heroin, hustling and homosexuality are the dominant features of their lives. Each hates men, each controls the hate with heroin, each hustles to get money to buy more heroin. Each *trick* increases their anger at the male sex. It's a truly vicious circle, with the fleeting friendship of their girlfriends their only basis for security.

I use the word fleeting because these girls have a life expectancy of thirty years of age with suicide, violence and overdosing with heroin being the common causes of their demise.

Criminal woman is certainly smarter than criminal man. In Canada, there is only one woman imprisoned to thirty-three men, and with a total national population of near sexual balance. One conclusion is that women are less criminal than men and let their men do the crime while they wait for the rewards. Another conclusion is that they are smarter and more devious.

Perhaps man in his law enforcement and trial duties is more lenient on the female offender. It can be argued that women's offences are less aggressive in type and do not require imprisonment because of the reduced social danger. Man's attitude in court appears tolerant and understanding if the woman commits what is considered to be a "female" crime. If she transgresses into man's aggressive criminal world as a bank robber, fraud organizer, or an emotional murderer, she is given the full weight of lawful sentence.

The fact that women generally have less physical strength than men furnishes only an indirect explanation of the specifity of female crimes, for it takes little strength to pull a trigger or handle burglar tools.

Women's crimes against the person include murder, infanticide, aggravated assault and false accusation. In the latter a vengeful woman may wrongfully accuse some man of a sexual attack.

Crimes against property include robbery and burglary, although the female is usually the accomplice decoy or driver. Theft, however, is the real domain and specialty of the female; shoplifting is a specifically female type of crime, with the modern theatre of operations being the department store and supermarket.

There are three different types of shoplifters. The "professional booster" travels from city to city on a scheduled plan. She steals articles, which she then sells to a *fence*, at discount prices, or to street friends who resell the articles for her. Her turnover is about $1,000 per working day. Then there is what I call the "necessary" thief. She maintains her family and herself in a comfortable lifestyle by stealing everything she needs – groceries, clothing, books, and indeed all of her Christmas and other gifts which she gets from very expensive stores.

The so-called respectable woman is in the third category with her shoplifting an extension of some mental torment and anger. She has no criminal interests, and usually no logical reason or need. I have known numerous women who have expressed their problems by "acquiring." One, a stable, well-employed woman, suddenly, without apparent reason, held up a furrier and attempted to leave the premises with an $8,000 mink coat. She was unmasked, had a plastic pistol and worked in a large company two blocks away. She did not want to work anymore and thought, illogically, that the robbery would solve that.

Another woman, the wife of a senior army officer, stole a pair of black leather gloves during the Christmas rush. She had been raised in England during the war years where queuing up had infuriated her. The Christmas line at the counter triggered an old playback emotional frustration and she left, taking the unpaid-for merchandise with her.

A third woman, again a professional, had shoplifted since adolescence. The crown attorney and her own counsel referred her to me prior to court. Raised by a penny-pinching father, she had been taught never to spend her money. Her father's axiom caused her to steal everything she needed. To give money away to a merchant was very disturbing to her. The treatment – pay for everything by cheque – solved her shoplifting problem

Fraud and false pretences are white collar professions, both in females and males. Minor frauds are the product of ingenious minds. One of Canada's leading banks lost $275,000 through fraud in the late 1960's. A quiet-natured bank teller was able, over a period of three years, to remain undetected – with an operational scheme so clever, that bank inspectors could not determine how the funds were disappearing. They knew the exact amounts of the monthly deficits, but nothing could be traced.

An anonymous informant told the bank manager that Cathy had two apartments, drove a blue Cadillac and frequently flew to Las Vegas. After two months' surveillance, police, armed with a search warrant, entered her two abodes to find deposit stubs to two different banks and a wardrobe of expensive clothing, including various items of mink apparel. In court, the total amount of her bank accounts, assets and jewelry balanced the bank deficit. She received eight years for her trouble. The sale of her assets at public auction was well attended by the curious middle class who came for a bargain and to obtain, at whatever cost, a first-hand product of the criminal mind.

Cathy spent fifty-six months at the Prison for Women, where she was accepted with admiration. There were no disagreements, no complaints and no psychiatric problems. In prison, as in the bank, she was a low-profile, pliant person whose mind was always on her own pleasure.

An impressive array of criminologists, female and male, consider deceitfulness to be the outstanding characteristic of the female offender. They base their conclusions on woman's lesser physical strength which leads her to rely on indirect aggressive behavior. They deduce that woman grows up in a life of self-concealment of physiological and hygenic functions.

In my own experience, I cannot accept the theory of woman's deceitfulness as the basis of her criminal acts. I recall the words of a male fraud offender who kept coming back to prison because of his expensive tastes. He remarked, "Doctor, you have to use what's going for you at the moment." Perhaps the female uses what's going for her at the moment. I believe she does.

The population of the Prison for Women has different prestige levels. There are residents, room-and-boarders, couple groups and incidental offenders. The residents are doing long sentences, form a stable core of the inmate system and are usually prison-wise, cautious and, at times, matriarchal in their controls. The roomers-and-boarders look upon themselves as temporary residents and do not really adapt to the inmate culture. Usually they are doing from two to four years. They have been crime-involved since childhood, have spent much of their lives on probation or in reform schools, and are usually a nuisance to law enforcement. They are thieves who steal from homes and stores, are alcohol-dependant, have no skills and live with little motivation. With them are the short-timers of two to five years who take part in some criminal action, but are not looked upon as dangerous – just plain unlucky.

The repeaters, while losers over and over again, bring to inmates sophisticated reports about things on the outside. They have their street connections and usually are skilled in bringing contraband drugs and articles into the prison. They are low-profile and are not trouble makers.

Mixed into these three levels are ethnic groups whose members support each other. Canadian Indians, French-speaking and Black inmates have separate relationships which never break the prestige ranks. There is also a loose provinicial identification, particularly among people from British Columbia, Ontario and Québec.

Couples constitute about thirty per cent of the population. Coupling removes the sense of isolation and loneliness and is the basis of the prison maxim, "You can't do time alone." Coupling is essentially a marriage for companionship, warmth and protection and inmates playing the male role are distinguishable from those playing the female role.

The *butch*, or male partner, is identified by her physical characteristics. She is usually stocky with a masculine walk and wears loose-fitting slacks with a short-sleeved T-shirt. Her shoes are low-heeled and occasionally she wears a beanie hat over a male haircut. Her voice is low with an authoritative inflection. She has names tattooed on her arms. Her breasts are not pronounced and her clothing attempts to disguise the female contours and achieve a flattened look. The *butch* changes her name to suit her role. Jean becomes John, Theresa becomes Terry, Ronalda becomes Ron and, if the name has no variables, a new name is adopted like Sam, Pete, Joe or Drago.

There is no coercion in coupling. Each partner makes a binding decision, realizing that sexual gratification is a service which individuals perform for each other. In the changing currents of the prison, many "marriages" are unstable and fleeting. After a final dislocation, new mates may be alined.

While the "marriage" combination is obvious, there are many "friend" relationships which are loyal and consistent and do not face the conflicts stemming from sexual involvements. Sometimes street friends join each other in prison, and frequently prison friends return to face society together.

Body tattoos are a significant announcement of the relationships of friends and lovers. Tattooing in women is a self-supporting declaration of identity and consists of puncturing the skin in a desired pattern, name or figure, with a coloring material so that the pattern is indelibly fixed.

In a series of examinations of tattooing in the population, I interviewed and examined the skin figures of twenty inmates.

One twenty-three-year-old manslaughter case, doing ten years, was professionally tattooed, while on a drinking bout, with a four-inch red heart transfixed with a green ribbon inscribed Diane and Jack. On the inside of her right leg five inches above the knee, was a self-done ink tattoo with the initials H.S. On her right ankle on the outside were the initials L.V. These tattoos were momentos of past relationships.

A twenty-two-year-old assaultive inmate imprinted her own name, Brenda, in one-inch letters on her left forearm. Two dots under her watch band indicated her time at Galt Institution. Several other ink marks led to a right shoulder initial T.C. A two-inch tattoo, Andrea, on the inner side of her right breast indicated a past marriage loyalty. On the left leg, some inches above the ankle, was a star with Al lettered beside it.

Most tattoos are simply written by using a needle and moistened thread with cigarette ashes rubbed into the fibres. The thread is drawn through the skin, as if sewing a seam, to leave its trace marks.

All the inmates indicated the first tattoos were self-implanted at training school. Some wished them removed for social and cosmetic reasons, others asked for removal because new partners resented old tattoos. Friends may have their names tattooed on each other although couples never engage in cross-identification.

Tattooing in the female population is never a random choice and always represents a serious emotional attachment. It establishes some factual identification and permanent significance to their otherwise barren and frustrating existence.

Their social code is less inclusive than the male inmate code. Prison terminology is in less frequent usage. Being *on point* is a strictly female term describing anxiety and concern that something is going to happen.

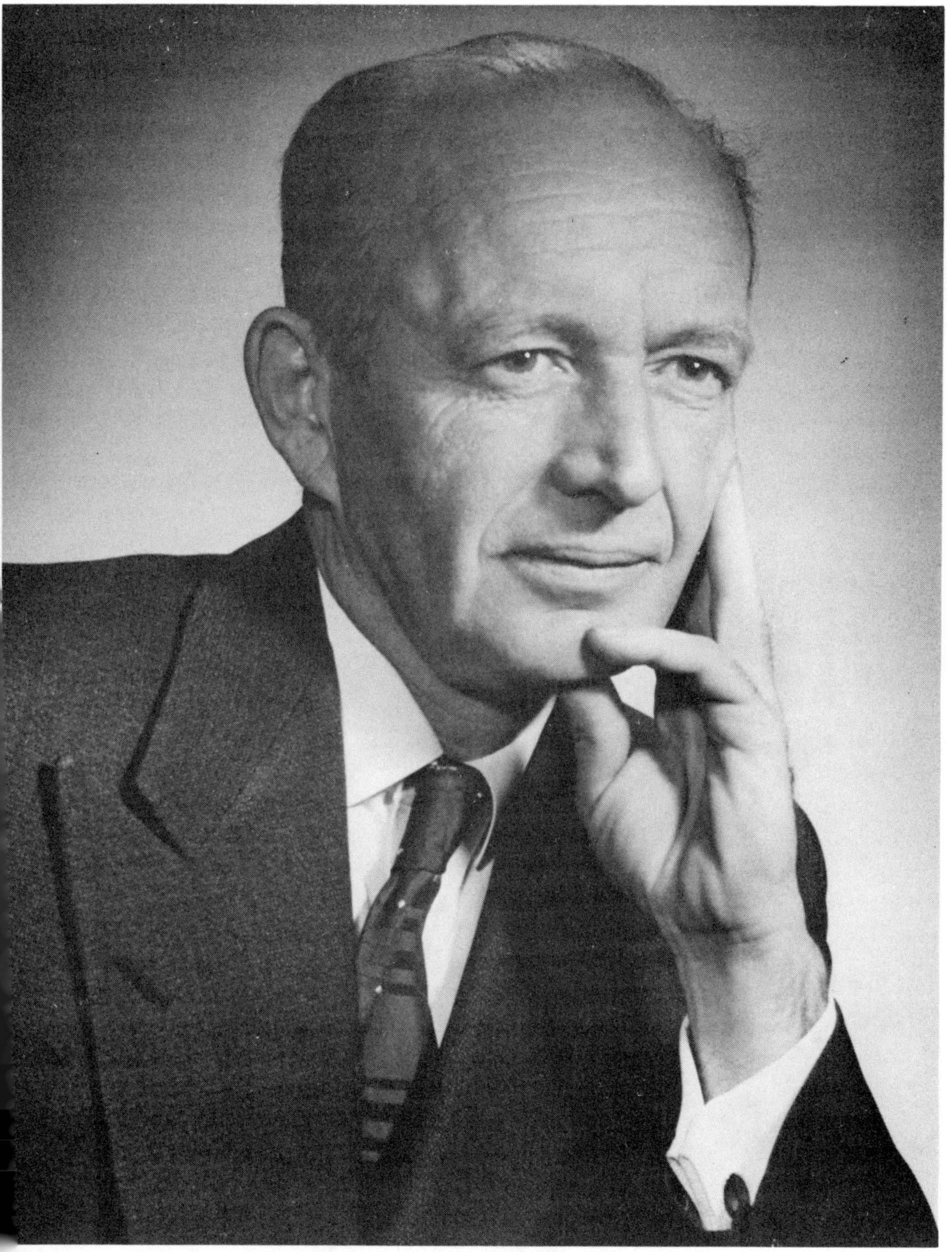

*r. Maurice O'Connor, 1910-1970, a pioneer in the field of psychiatry t Kingston Penitentiary from 1949-1958, was one of Canada's leading sychiatrists. He established the first psychiatric unit in the federal enitentiary system and introduced modern and progressive treatment chniques. He is particularly remembered for his scientific and umanistic approach to the inmate.*
*ourtesy of George Scott)*

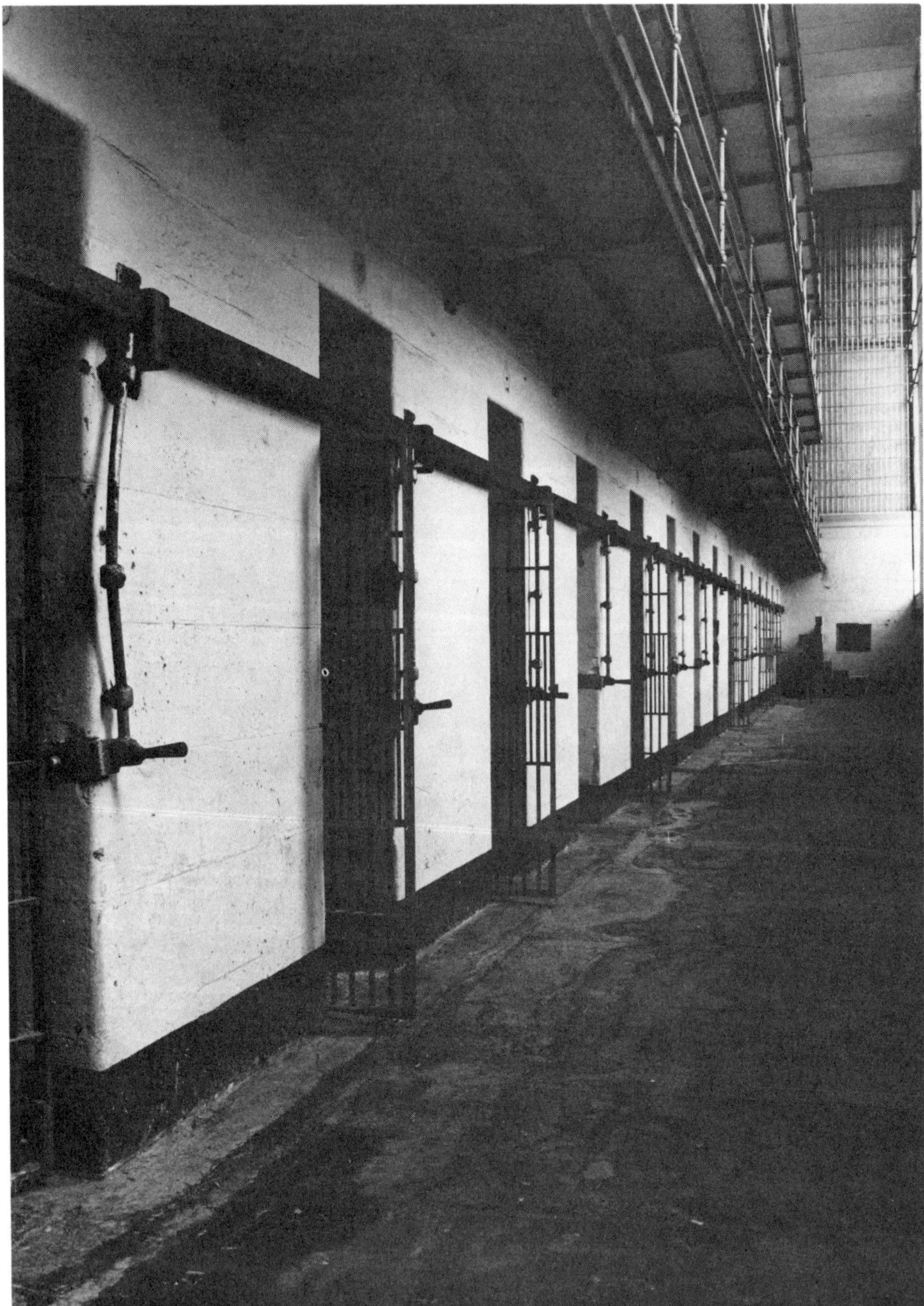

*A three-tiered cell block in the riot-torn area of Kingston Penitentiary (1971). The upright bar near the far-left cell, was forced free by rioting inmates who murdered its occupant – a sex offender.*
*(Kingston Whig-Standard)*

*A dinner fork, with a few twists and bends, can become a dangerous weapon. It is designed for personal protection rather than for purposes of assault.*
*(Courtesy of George Scott and the Kingston Penitentiary medical department)*

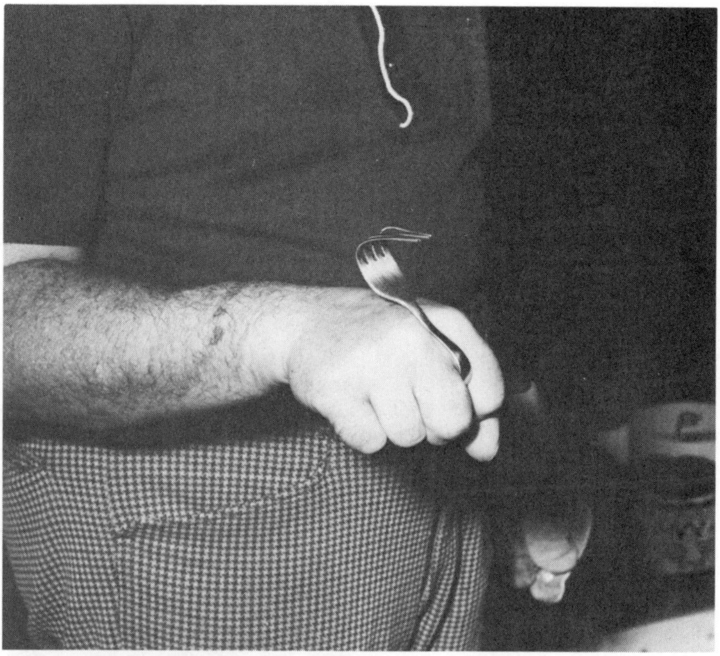

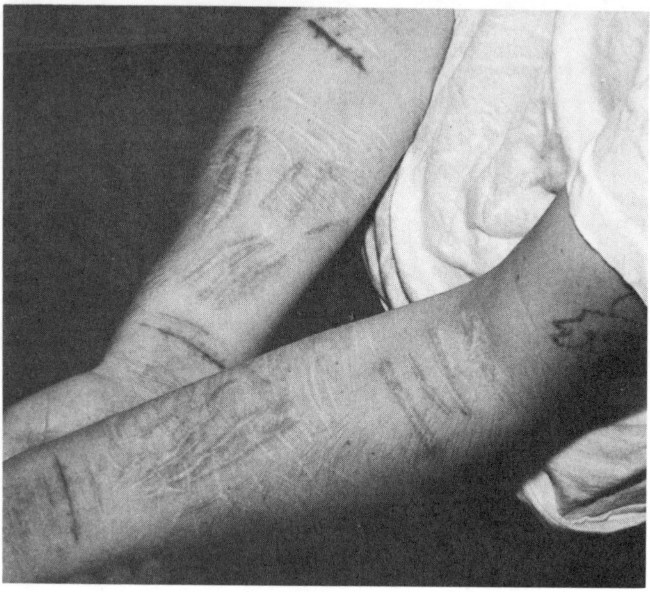

*Slashing is not an uncommon occurrence in the prison population. New scars are superimposed on older faded scars on both arms, indicating that this prisoner has expressed his pent-up anger and resentment on two separate occasions.* *(Barry Wright)*

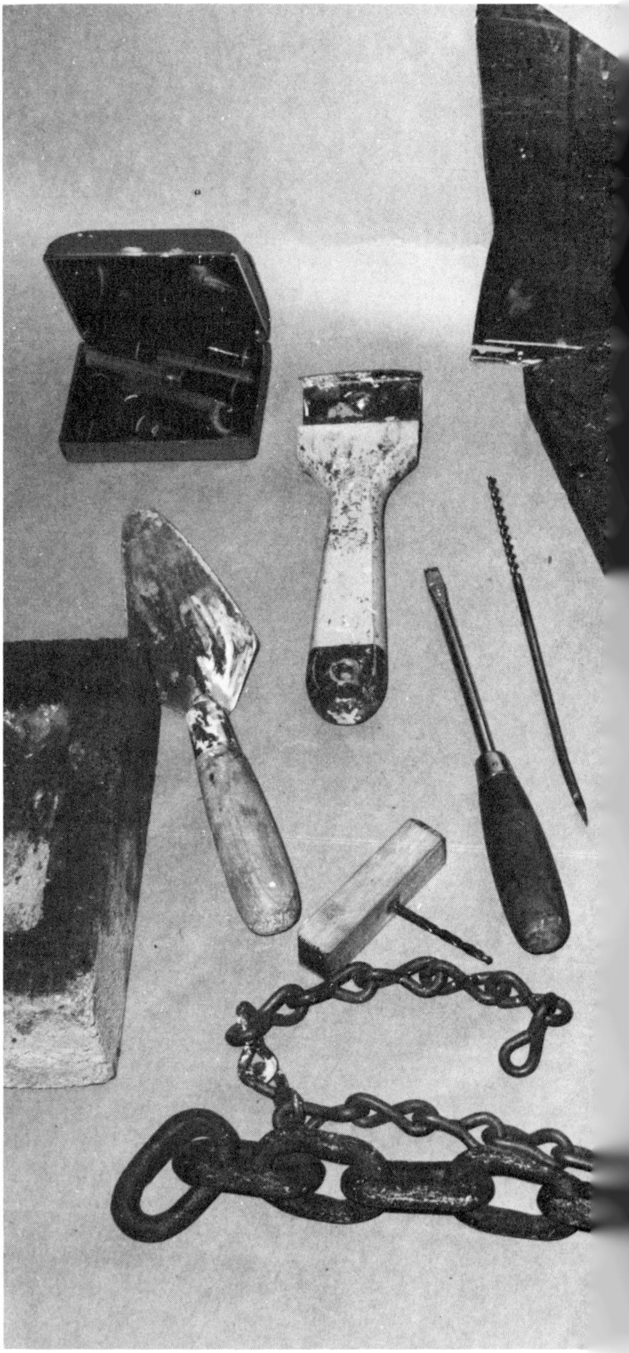

*Routine searches of inmate cells yield a wide variety of contraband, which may include street money, food and pills. Hand-fashioned weapons, such as the twenty-three shown here, are the most common items discovered.*

*(Barry Wright)*

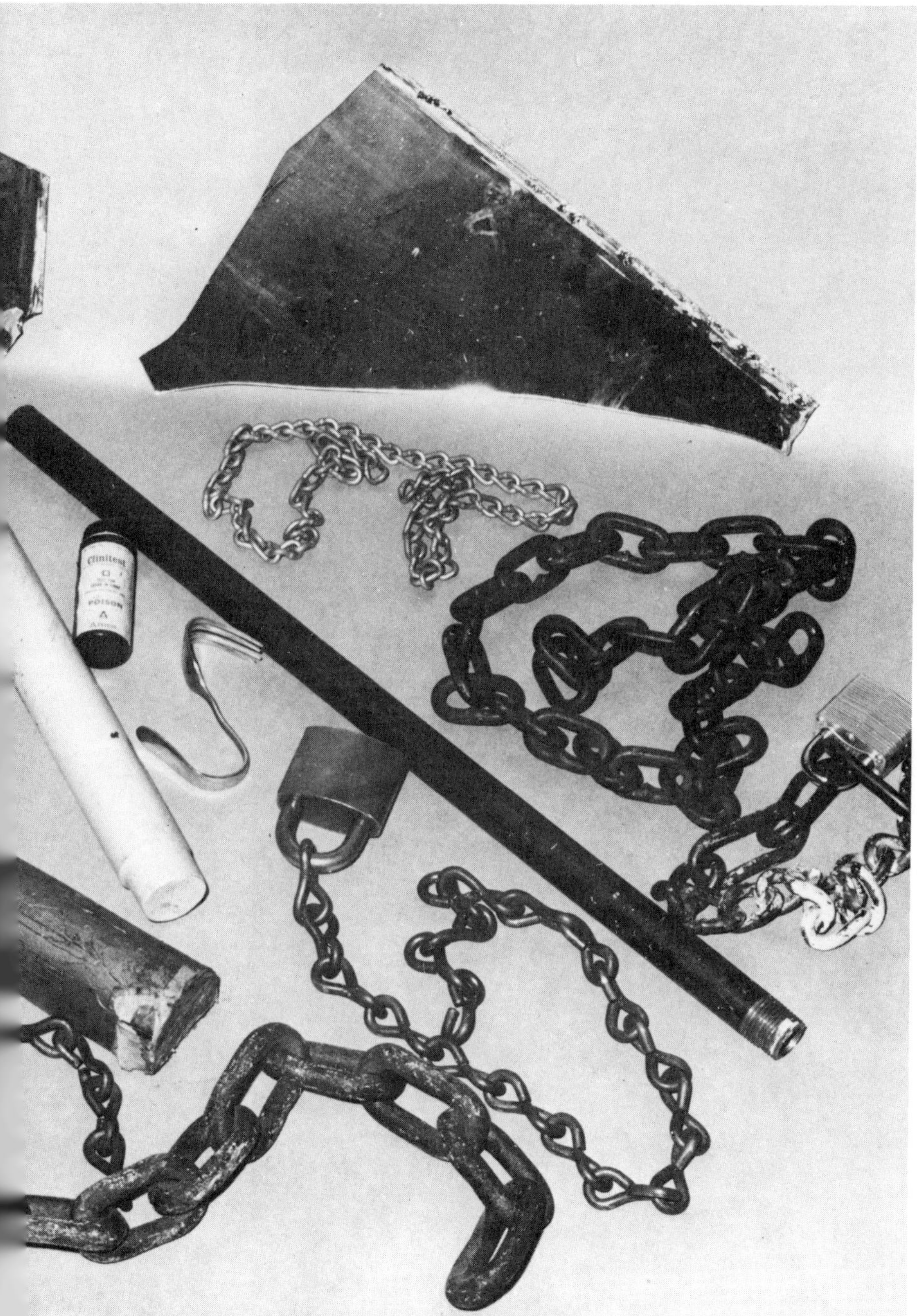
Clinitest
POISON

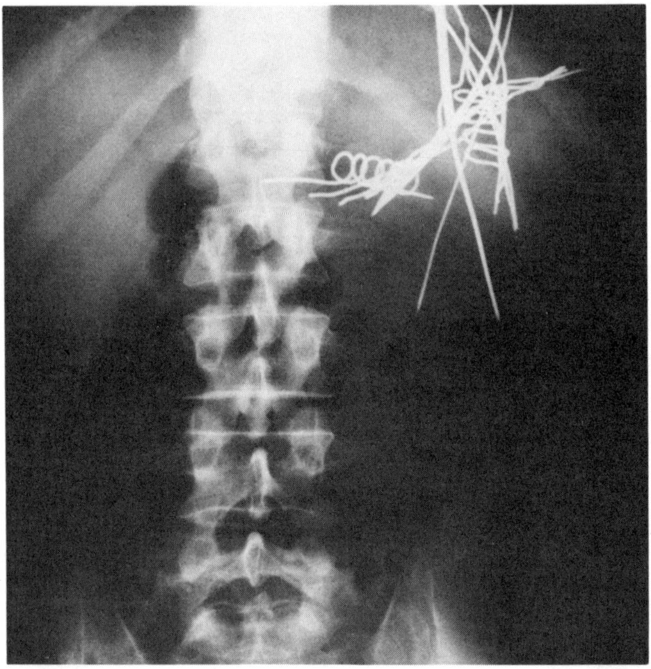

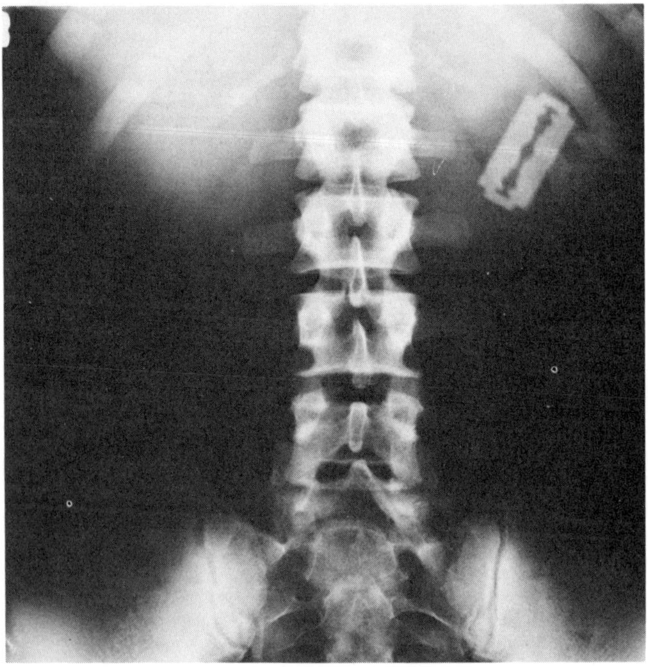

*Swallowing foreign objects is a bizarre and infrequent method of gaining attention and is always considered to be crucial.*
*(upper left) copper wire*
*(lower left) razor blade*
*(upper right) bent fork*
*(lower right) five spoon handles*

*(Courtesy of George Scott the Kingston Penitentiary medical department)*

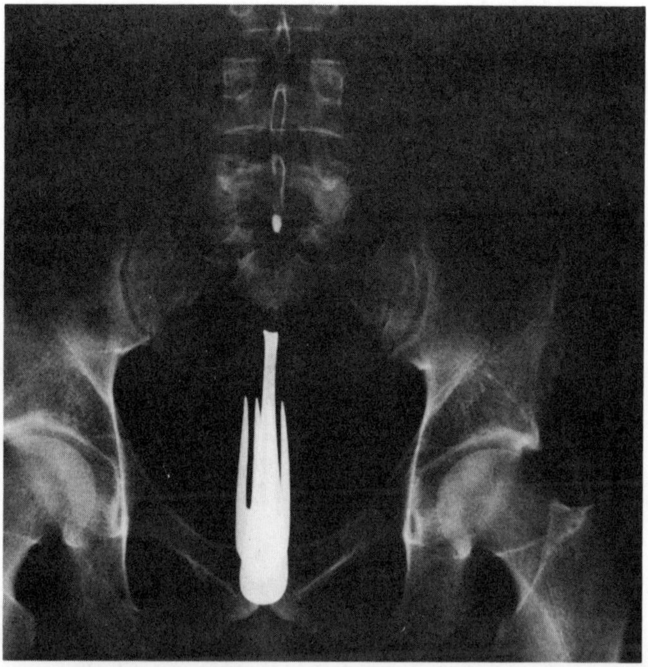

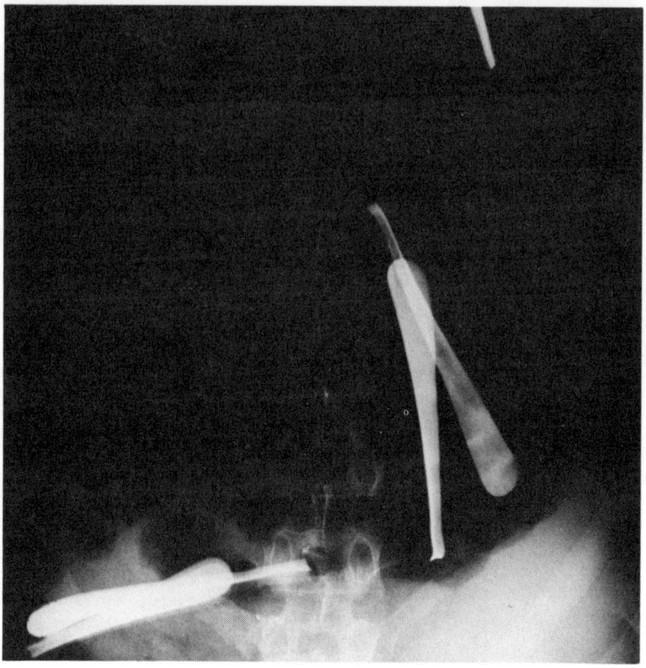

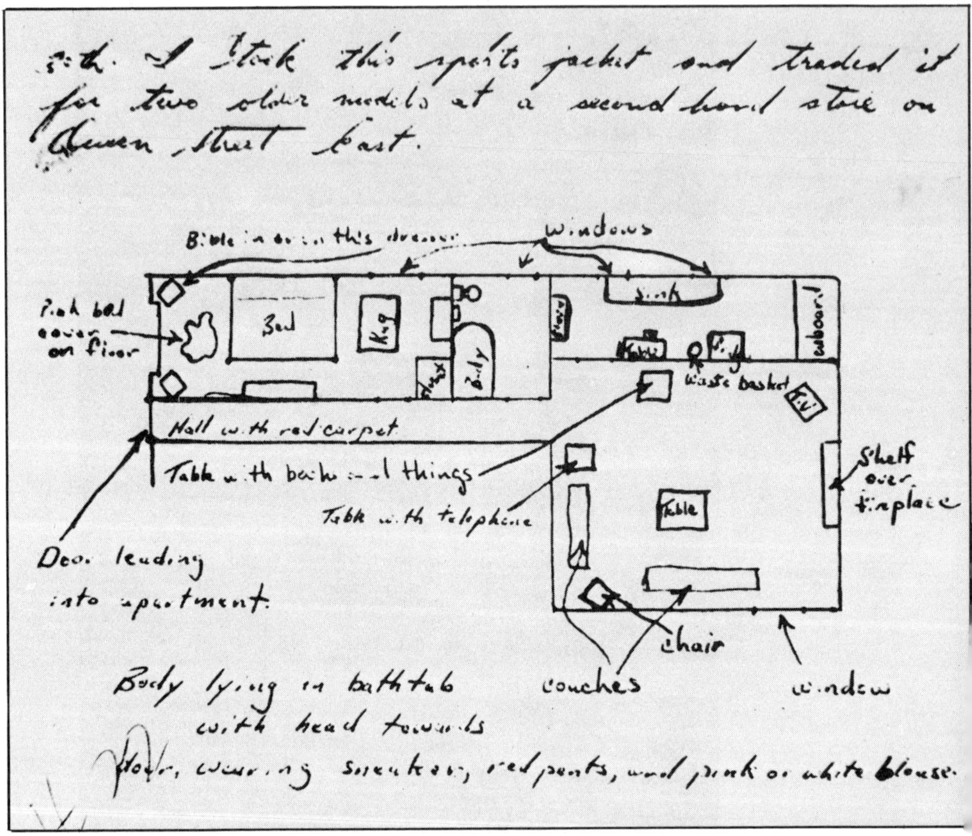


An inmate's accurate and detailed drawing to support his confession of the undetected murder of a Toronto woman.

(Courtesy of George Scott and the Kingston Penitentiary medical department)

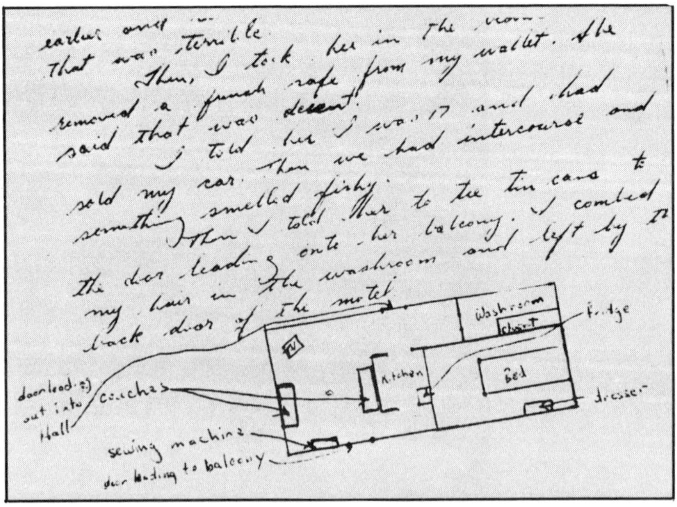


A false confession, which the same inmate gave to me over a period of months.

Females are more compassionate in reporting expected suicides and notifying the staff that certain factions are declaring war.

The sanctions against stealing and debts are universal in the system. An inmate who has been a known police informant, particularly for the R.C.M.P., has an uneasy time throughout her sentence and usually withdraws to segregation. Certain offenders whose crimes relate to child abuse, indecent assaults and contributing to delinquency are isolated and treated with contempt. Although specific occurrences of violence are uncommon, the killing of a drug peddler or a kinky, perverted patron of prostitution, is seen as commendable and assures acceptance into the prison society. Females who meddle in others' personal affairs and ridicule couples and friends face sudden physical violence at any time, as do inmates who attempt to break up relationships.

Females who manage to form relationships with male staff are given great praise – in return for details of the "action." While men are hated in principle, they are good subjects for an involvement effort. In fact, any man who functions in a relationship with the inmates feels the pressure of their presence, for better or worse. On two occasions, male staff have emerged from the scene with hurt pride, damaged egos and loss of effectiveness.

Psychiatry in a women's prison is a daily exercise in compromise. It is double-edged because psychiatric skills have to bow to the more impelling force of inmate survival and the inmates have to compromise their needs into a funnel of psychiatric usefulness. Women inmates see psychiatry in a more personalized manner than do their male counterparts. Some come to ask for help in understanding their offences, others wish to understand what keeps "bringing me back." Women look upon the psychiatrist with respect because they feel he functions at the level of a con man and, win or lose, there are no hard feelings. Occasionally, however, differences occur which are neither predictable, nor debatable.

On one occasion, Denise was referred to me to assess her suitability for a day pass to downtown Kingston without an escort. She sat down without a word and looked icily at me. She was about five foot seven in height, with a style and manner worthy of a second glance. Her high heels indicated a special occasion as did her loosely buttoned blouse. Her hands restlessly fingered a plastic ashtray. She appeared to be waiting for something. I couldn't catch her glance and asked, "Denise, what's burning you up?"

There was no response. She was obviously angry.

"Let's talk about the day pass," I said.

"You can take it and stuff it," she said, "I don't want no pass."

And then the storm broke. Up she stood and with a circular motion of her arms cleaned the desk top. Calendar, books, blotter and pencil holder, all disappeared to the right. Next the plastic ashtray flew past my head as I arose from the chair (a chair is a hell of a place to be caught in). Denise took two steps back to the window ledge and let fly a pot of geraniums which glanced off my left shoulder and splattered into fragments against the wall.

Around my desk she came, breathing violence and anger. I met her straight on and wrapped my arms around her waist. She was unable to strike me or scratch me, but was bent on biting me. My right arm around her waist moved automatically to grasp her long black hair. With a tug I flipped her off balance and with a noisy thud she struck the floor like a sack of potatoes. There I was, standing astride of her. She was motionless. She looked at me with a meaningless stare then closed her eyes.

By this time the nurse and custodial officer arrived. "Are you all right Doctor Scott?"

"Yes, I'm O.K.," I said, "but you'd better help Denise. I think she's a bit damaged."

With help she got to her feet and walked slowly over the geraniums and down the hall to the health care office where she remained for some twenty minutes. I visited her later and she exploded: "Scott, where in the hell did you get that move? You must have worked in a slaughter-house." She was fuming."O.K. George, the next time I get out, I'll shoot both your kneecaps off. Mark my words."

It's difficult to follow conventional psychiatric practices in prison. Women inmates require listening time so that they can talk about their tensions and problems. There is always an emotional component of dependency in their actions. Inmates carefully monitor those going to psychiatry as to time and frequency. Patients consult with each other on the techniques most effective in obtaining sedative medications.

If the psychiatrist spends too much time, there is a basis for conjecture. "She's working him" someone will say, or "He's conned into her gag." Yet, from time to time, sincerely motivated inmates receive valuable psychotherapy, with increased understanding of stress areas and coping techniques. New long-term arrivals come for support and advice. Bizarre and unique offenders establish psychiatric relationships to convince the population that their crimes were because of mental reasons. Others seek answers for their dangerousness.

One such example, Jill, was the centre of psychiatric study for some twenty-three sessions. She received life for the murder of her boyfriend. She had been in court for murder of a similar nature two years previously, but was acquitted on the basis that she was so drunk she didn't know what she was doing. In all events, she murdered the second man, an individual of similar build and temperament, with a knife wound in exactly the same location as the first one, and strangely enough, in a similar state of drunkeness. The victim had been told by friends to keep away from Jill or he'd end up like her earlier friend.

Jill, aged twenty-six, buxom with red hair and freckles, strong brown eyes and a faint Scottish accent, was greatly concerned about her future and had more than the usual comments about her judge and trial. I involved myself in her detailed history and as the thirteenth member of the jury began to weigh the probabilities of her statements. As no weapon was found, and as Jill was amnesic for the critical hours, I was curious about her memory loss. I used a conventional pentothal analysis to reduce her controls and added an anaesthetic gas, nitrous oxide (laughing gas), to excite her dormant memories. The treatment went on for some forty-five weeks, each alternate session being an analysis session. Jill, although in a deep state of drowsiness, rolled back her amnesic areas slowly and eventually was able to review all her actions except for a critical five-minute period.

"I went to another room to get undressed and the next thing I remember was putting a pillow under Robert's head and covering him with a blanket," she said. "I didn't have a knife." She indicated that a second male acquaintance may have killed her friend, knowing that, when drunk, she was amnesic.

I have known Jill for fifteen years. She is overweight, suffers from high blood pressure, and is given to alcohol and drug dependency. Her life sentence is a true life sentence as she will in all likelihood die some coming night from the accumulated emotional and physical traumas in her life. Jill cannot handle the streets and if she did go out, would use alcohol until it killed her.

She is frank, outspoken, profane and human. Both inmates and custodial officers are fond of her and certainly both pamper her.

* * *

Everyone has a most unforgettable person in his past. I have one and I call her Violet. I've known her for twenty years. I don't really know if she is unforgettable, or unforgivable. Someone else has to be the judge of that. Certainly she created an impression on everyone with whom she came into contact.

I first met her at the Prison for Women when she was nineteen. She reminded me of the bobbysoxers of the day, with pale, knobby knees and toed-in legs. Her body was boy-like. Her face was a study of childhood mischief, a dimpled chin below a rather wide mouth. Her blue eyes looked you up and down and then over your shoulder. She certainly could engage anyone, though no one could engage her. She never got angry and never used swear words. You couldn't condone the many troublesome moments she caused people. Yet, I kept reminding myself, how you can reject a life-sized raggedy doll with blue eyes, waving arms and toes like that?

It was 1961 when Violet arrived at the Prison for Women, not on a real criminal charge but for escaping from a training school. And today, no one talks about the institution without mentioning her name.

Violet is a kind of symbol of the prison – a reminder of all the kids who went wrong and ended up on the junk pile. And there have been a good many of them over the years. She could be cute and pixie-like, sometimes lovable and sometimes not, but her usual adolescent sweetness masked the vinegar barrel from which she emerged.

Violet was the youngest of four children. Her father, Rick, was a night watchman at a hotel. Working all night and sleeping all day, he had little time for the children. Violet's mother, Helen, wasn't exactly what you'd call family-oriented. In fact, she spent as little time as possible with the young ones.

Violet was six when Helen began taking an interest in her. Her mother thought she should have a trade and began giving her lessons in shoplifting.

"Violet," Helen instructed her at the start, "place the pack of cards between your knees and walk around the kitchen without dropping them."

Helen applauded her daughter's first efforts.

"Now tomorrow night, you'll practise going up and down the stairs. When you steal from a department store, you won't always be on the ground floor."

Mother's next lesson was to have Violet wear her jacket with one sleeve filled with crushed paper and a glove, filled with facial tissue, sewn to the sleeve. Her own arms and hands were free across her waist inside the jacket. This exercise was directed at stealing articles close to the counter edge.

The following lesson involved stealing rings, earrings and other trinkets: "Just swallow them, honey, and Old Helen will get them for you later."

Then there was the raincoat trick for rainy days. Through a long slash, the girl could stash away records, boxes of chocolates and similar things. Helen had even sewn pockets on the inside of the coat especially for groceries and meat.

In school, Violet developed terrorist tactics. She blocked toilets, emptied lunch boxes, scattered snowboots and other clothing. Sometimes she let the air out of the tires of the teachers' cars.

Eventually she was expelled, but her nuisance tactics continued. She would telephone teachers' wives with gossip. Then she would phone women teachers and tell them of each other's adulteries, all of the stories, of course, being fabrications.

Helen became annoyed when her daughter began playing tricks on her. It wasn't funny to be told, by a serious, earnest voice that your husband had just been in a fatal accident, or that a daughter had just been arrested. Helen went to the school for help. Soon after, a truant officer visited Violet. Declared a truant, she was taken to court where she was judged to be delinquent and sent to the Galt Training School for Girls.

Galt.

Violet scoffed. All those stupid girls and all those kooky guards. It was not long before she escaped, crossed the border at Detroit and hitchhiked to Atlanta. There, at a service station, she drove off with the owner's car. Back in Canada later, she told a tall story of being kidnapped on the street in Galt.

Some time later, she was missing again from the training school. This time she spent two weeks in Toronto, stealing electrical utensils from the big stores and selling them to a fence she had found. She had $160 in her pocket when the police caught up with her, but they just figured she had been soliciting and sent her back to Galt.

Her third escape did not turn out too well. She stole from a casual acquaintance she met at a bar. He punched her in the face, dragged her into his car and dumped her off in the country without shoes to walk in. Arrested for escaping, she was sent this time to the Prison for Women.

In prison she teamed up as a couple with a flat-chested inmate, becoming a *butch* for a spell but she had no interest, nor even awareness, of sex in any form whatever.

She was given educational courses and library privileges but these didn't change things. After a year, she told me, she could go out on the street and make a good living *boosting* from electrical appliance stores.

Violet did not lose her desire for escape at the prison. The first time she donned an offier's uniform and simply walked out of the front door with a friend. They spent two weeks in Ottawa and then were returned. She got an extra two years for her escapade.

Soon after, she arranged to see a specialist at a general hospital and escaped en route. This time she spent six weeks in Montreal. Another two-year sentence was meted out.

In a third escape she took an officer hostage, released her and took off in a prison car, which ran out of gas thirty-five miles away. Again she was given extra time to serve.

Eight years after she entered the Prison for Women, she was a pudgy, twenty-seven-year-old woman with a drawn smile and faded eyes, a tragically lonely individual who still managed to keep some of the old spark alive.

She finally was allowed day parole and spent two weekends at the home of a female custodial officer. On the second visit, she stole the woman's car and travelled to British Columbia and back. Returning the car to its owner she said, with a shrug of the shoulders, that she was sorry.

Violet was probably one of the few females who could lay claim to the title of con artist. When she zeroed in on something she wanted, she usually got it. She always seemed to have something cooking on all four burners and yet somewhere in all that scheming machinery there still existed a mischievous little girl.

She had the undeniable appeal of the small girl who would grin and say, "Can I bum a smoke?" or "You got any gum?" or "Can you tell me what's going on around here? I won't tell anybody else." It was hard to realize, as you looked into those eyes and saw that grin, that you were talking to a seasoned inmate who had spent three-quarters of her life incarcerated, and knew every trick in the book.

Violet's life is still pulsating. She is out there now, free. Somewhere. I don't know where. Some day she'll call me, I'm sure. In the meantime I hope nobody hurts her as she goes down her chosen road. She is too much of an expert at hurting herself.

**CHAPTER 18**

# Michael and Sean Were Sweethearts

Michelle slips easily out of the back seat of the police car this blustery fall day and draws her coat close to ward off the cold. Under sheriff's escort, she walks the few steps to the main door of the Prison for Women, pauses as though to savor free air for the last time and enters.

She is a svelte young woman with medium brown hair and bright, sharp eyes. The eyes, in fact, are the most striking features of her attractive face. She is put through the usual formalities and officially admitted as an inmate. Later, she is taken into the privacy of the senior matron's office.

She is starting a three-year stretch for helping her boyfriend escape from a Toronto jail and for participating in an armed robbery afterwards – but it's not her criminal record that comes up in the interview.

"I'm concerned about you being here," the matron says.

Michelle shrugs.

"Weren't you a prisoner at Collins Bay (the male penitentiary) about three years ago?"

"Yeah," Michelle says in a low voice.

"The reports from Toronto indicate you've had..." the matron stops to clear her throat, "...that you've had the operation...the sex operation...and that you are now recognized as a woman. Is this so?"

"Yes, it is."

"I hope you're all right here." There is a note of seriousness in the matron's voice. "Security will give you a fair shake but you'll have to be careful. With your new sex, the butches may really take a fancy to you." She pauses and laughs. "You're the first man to be admitted to the Prison for Women, you know. Well, the first changed man."

In the annals of Canadian crime, the story of Michelle and her boyfriend Sean, holds a unique place. Sean fell in love with Michelle, certain that she was a girl. When he found out that Michelle was really a boy, and that her name was Michael however, he continued the love affair.

But let's look back over the years.

Michael was an only son with five older sisters. His father treated him "like the rest of the girls," as the record indicates. Michael was slight in build, with a gentle manner and a soft, shy voice. He seemed to fit into his sisters' lives (the closest was ten years his senior), listening to them, following their romances with boyfriends. At school, he was an average student but he had no time for classmates, refused to take part in athletics and would not use the school bathrooms. By the age of thirteen, he was wearing girls' slacks and loafers and had let his hair grow down to his shoulders. By this time, too, male classmates were making him uncomfortable with rude and degrading remarks.

Michael's adjustment posed a difficult problem and after entreating his parents, he was allowed to stay with his sister, May, a clerk typist in a downtown office, who became his best friend. She enrolled her brother in a night course at a nearby high school but, realizing that he thought and acted like a girl, she had him inscribed as a female. For three years, he attended classes dressed in jeans and sweater (with under puffs to swell his breasts). When he graduated it was as a female – though he still possessed an unwanted penis and testicles.

At seventeen, Michael, now calling himself Michelle, met Sean, a young taxi driver who occasionally drove 'her' to work at an insurance company. Sean thought from the beginning that Michelle wasn't like other girls but it was only after several anxious dates that he became aware of her genital variation. Instead of abusing her, he simply said "You've got too much baggage." To that he added, moments later, "But you're still my girl."

Over the months, Sean protected him and, in a gentle way, guided him through the maze of problems that face the transverse, or transsexual, male. He read all he could about sex changes and at the height of their romance, promised him he would find out about the sex change operation.

Seven thousand dollars was out of sight in the taxi business – but there were alternatives. The couple decided to go on a robbery spree. They did, were arrested and each given a five-year sentence. Details of their experiences at Collins Bay were somewhat tortuous but nothing changed their unique relationship. Michelle shaved every day, but otherwise maintained a ladylike poise and dignity in standard male prison garb. Sean's burly appearance and brusque manner discouraged comments from the curious population.

I saw Michael, or Michelle, on two occasions and decided the speech, mannerisms, and even appearance were those of a woman. Within twenty-eight months, Michelle returned to Toronto on parole, with Sean following four months later. They moved into a small apartment and Sean returned to the taxi business.

They staged several other robberies and collected $5,000. Then, one night, Tim drove her to a movie and went on to work. The next morning he was in court charged with assault causing bodily harm. He was given two nine-year sentences.

Michelle remained in Toronto while Sean sat out his time at Collins Bay. By careful saving, Michelle managed to augment their robbery-gotten gains to $7,000. He then went to the Gender Clinic of the Clarke Institute and had the operation, which was carried out without complications. During the ensuing year, Michelle followed the post-surgical program carefully and, in effect, became totally female.

There was, however, a problem. An ex-inmate may not visit an inmate of a federal prison. Some time later, Sean was taken to a Kingston hospital for minor surgery and Michelle engineered a plan to pick him up in a car as he emerged from the building. The escape went well but within two hours the couple was apprehended on Highway 401 east of Port Hope. Sean had an extra two years added to his sentence and Michelle was sent to the Prison for Women as a result of this escapade.

Michelle was released from prison in June 1979, and is now employed as an operator of a small store in Hamilton – and, with the most astounding loyalty, is waiting for Sean to make it to the street.

Sexuality – it's the crucible of life. Our very beings depend on the sexuality of others. It develops future generations. Yet, is sexuality a mental complex, an emotional one, a physical one, or all of these? Is sexuality a simple response to biological sensors existing in each human?

Sexuality in our culture is expected to function within appreciated boundaries. Mates, according to script, must be of similar height. Males must be two to five years older than their female partners. Body figures have to be typed in similar casts: pudgy, athletic, slim. Partners must not come from different skin cultures.

Age becomes a pathological factor whenever one member of a couple is fifteen or twenty years older than the other. If the male is older, someone is bound to say, "He's old enough to be her father." If the woman is the older one, someone likely will tell the man that his lady friend is old enough to be his mother.

The concept of parallel types – tall with tall, athletic with athletic and so on – supposedly paves the way for a successful marriage. To breach the law of similarities is to break an unspoken, primitive covenant, the survival of the species. Yet, while the physical similarities are obvious, the emotionality of each partner is the real pyramid basis for the relationship.

Relationships in courting and mating are modified so that excesses of impulsive anger, bitter profanity and overt cupidity are hidden. One must now show one's temperament variations. Since romantic periods have to be romantic but marriages do not, the later life may produce some unexpected developments.

In some cases, a man's romantic and restrained sexuality impresses his bride-to-be. A gentle, soft-spoken groom with no obvious sexual preoccupation and an apparent consideration for women may well impress a woman. On the other hand, his restrained sexuality may also be due to an aversion to the female sex. He may be a developmental homosexual who manages to function at the margin of masculinity.

I speak of variations in sexuality in terms of degrees of awareness of sexual opposites at a party or gathering. Men, as a group, have a seductive interest in women of their age or younger. At a party, for instance, they are apt to make a play for some woman, yet on a personal basis, have no desire to accompany her when she leaves the group.

Women are not seductive in broadcast fashion. They more likely will be selective in terms of one particular male. One young lady I know makes the point very clearly. She first observed her husband-to-be in a lab where he was working on a chemistry experiment. "I knew at a glance I would marry him," she recalls, "and at the time I didn't even know his name." The mating impulse has strong evidence to support the claim that it is beyond rational control. It is not uncommon for a man and a woman to have a striking emotional awareness preceding verbal communication. "I feel I've known you for years!" is an oft-repeated exclamation.

Sexual identity has components of bio-genetic vitality (hereditary factors), developmental identification (personal experience) and circumstantial responses (personal needs).

Bio-genetic vitality refers to the genetic ordinates of both parents, which have paired into a biological being. These ordinates have the male and female rudiment structures which develop together for several weeks of fetal life.

As genetic dominance is established in the chromosomal family, the male and female differential is made. Although nature is designed for perfection, a delay in the genetic differentiation may give days of parallel growth to embryonic internal sex systems. Further delays in sex determination may cause serious problems. At the end of the scale, a person may well be born with the combined features of both male and female, a condition we call the "hermes-aphrodite mix."

The mix can produce a structured male whose features, habits and mannerisms indicate a female host inside. On the other hand, a female may have the complete physical assemblage of her sex and yet have biochemical traits and certain mannerisms indicating there is a man host inside her.

The second level of sexual identification occurs in the long process of developmental identification. The critical relationship here is between the child and his parents, aunts, uncles, teachers and friends. A boy raised in a broken home with a critical, paranoid mother, two older sisters who belittle him and female teachers who correct and discipline him, will develop a hurtful image of all women. Regarding the female domain as antagonistic, he may develop comfortable relationships with his male teacher, or sports coach. I remember one man who told me very plainly, "I hate women. All women. I hate their voices, their clothes, their perfume. And with sex, they don't turn me on." There is no doubt that rejection by the opposite sex produces varying degrees of caution and immaturity in inter-sexual relationships.

The developmental tragedy in girls is more damaging than that in the male. While small boys may be damaged by overwhelming females, little girls suffer devious sexual exploitation at the hands of their fathers, uncles, brothers and male neighbors.

These little girls may suffer genital manipulation on a frequent basis as the male attempts to arouse an erotic response. They soon learn that their fathers, uncles or brothers are doing something wrong, particularly if they are given money and told not to say anything. By adolescence, these girls have no warm sensitivity about men. They become man-defensive for their entire lives so it is little wonder they choose women for friends. In the course of their lives, they exert effort to destroy predatory man operating around them. It is easy to understand why young prostitutes have no feeling for sexual encounters. They realize that now they can exploit men who, in their defenceless years, exploited them.

Both these groups, by rejecting their sexual opposites, resort exclusively to relationships with their own sex, for comfort, company, affection and sexual enjoyment. Perhaps the gay world is actually gay, happy and carefree because its adherents have attained freedom from the domineering, castigating opposite sex.

Circumstantial responses are those sexual attitudes and tones that develop out of everyday experience. In situations where a couple has been separated because of employment or illness, or where the partners simply have not been able to relate sexually, the male may regress to less mature mechanisms. He may make sly attempts at dating, read girlie books, become a park-peeper, or seek other sexual substitutions.

Many seemingly normal males, under stress, return to the adolescent adherence to the male and may become active in transient homosexual activities. Some slip deeper into sexual infantalism with self-satisfying habits of overeating, oversleeping and masturbation.

The involved variations in sexual life, identification and maladjustment stem from readily identifiable sources. It is obvious that criminal man is not born criminal but in early life has been exposed to harmful, traumatic, inconsistent care. He then is more prone to reflect sexual maladjustment. Criminal woman, more so even than the man, shows the overwhelming scars of sexual injury.

In prison, these multi-damaged personalities try to keep a sexual balance in accord with their environment. Behind bars, sexuality is never discussed at the administrative level. It lies quietly and totally within the sphere of inmate life. Sexual isolation is the primary complication of the prison experience.

Man's sexual patterns in society contain irradiated forms of voyeurism, fetishism, exhibitionism and other *isms*. Man also goes for massage parlor treatments, mate swapping, homosexual tearooms, burlesque, and blue movies. The complicated world of sexual expression, however, is altered markedly in the prison experience.

Behind the walls, the individual lives in isolation from the opposite sex, is usually fearful that his sexual interests will disapppear and struggles to keep his sexuality activated. Some prisoners are able to reject sexual interests. The usual inmate, however, attempts to establish his program of sexual activity either by himself, or with a partner. Sexuality may become overt in nature in that forced sex becomes a reinforcement of masculinity.

Sexual assaults are not homosexual attacks but assaults by heterosexual males on other males to show power and dominance. Victims are degraded, humiliated and forced into the role of the passive partner. The purpose is to have a number of terrified, humiliated males available in the population to satisfy the needs of the controlling males. The frightened, degraded men usually are quick to respond to such commands as "Bend over," or "Grab your ankles."

From time to time, the *daddys*, as they are called, use the gentle approach, singling out a younger prisoner because of his youth and build. They may protect their "boys" and give them gifts in exchange for sexual favors. The usual procedures here are oral, genital, fellatio and anal intercourse. Simpler erotic experiences involve mutual masturbation, called a *handshake*; and *legging*, the act of reaching ejaculation by inserting the male organ between the legs of a cooperating male.

There is a curtain of silence concerning sexual activity in the prison world. I have talked to many inmates over the years and, without exception, they were all embarrassed about my inquiries. "Everybody does his own thing," one inmate told me. Another, a thirty-year-old lifer, said, "There's nothing kinky going on. We stop anything that smacks of force. What sex goes on, goes on when it's O.K. for both." I asked still another man about masturbation. "It's for the kids," he replied.

"For us older guys, it's anal intercourse. Between friends, that's all right."

The inmates who are most likely to seek psychiatric help are the effeminate ones. They are known as *queens* and their hair, voices and mannerisms are feminine.

"I've been hurt so many times," one of the *queens* said to me not long ago. "I can't think about it because it hurts so much." As he talked, I tried to see in him the gay sexual player at age twenty. His face was lined and drawn, his voice hushed and halting, and instinctively I knew his sexual life has involved many male opportunists who used him for fellational adventures.

At forty, he had spent half of his life in prison – but that is the way he wanted it. "There's nothing on the street for me," he confided. "I always like to get back to jail where I know everybody and where everything is nice."

Every man carries in his mind scattered remnants of pain and hate and, no matter the context, he cannot be divorced from his animal brothers. Sexual domination is an animal attribute, and in the primitive recesses of social man are tempered and modified sexual compulsions. Arousal in itself is random response to the presence of an accepting female.

In all cases, sexual aggression is directed toward domination of the female, who is placed in a subservient role. Rape returns man to his primitive behavior and, in context, is the random aggressive subjugation of the female. Rape is precipitated, not through affability and seductivity, but by circumstances which awaken the insular remnants of hate and pain which women have inflicted upon him. Man is particularly weighted to rape if he has an overwhelming degree of frustration toward his wife, girlfriends, mother or sister, which he is unable to express. Alcohol and provocation frequently lower his controls, producing a violent, impulsive sexual act devoid of human feelings.

I have had a great many interviews with rapists and there is a pattern to their comments. These are some of them:

"I hate all the women in my life because they have hurt me."

"I suddenly hate this woman because something in her has aroused angry memories from the past."

"I could never strike my mother as she is a woman."

"I can't strike this woman because I'd never do that to any woman."

But the rapist makes it clear that he doesn't have to strike a woman. He has an alternative. Here are two comments from my notepads:

"I'll express my anger in a violent blow to her sexuality."

"I won't hit her. I'll just show her that, as a woman, she can't punish me anymore. I'll show her I can dominate her."

Indecent assault is a less direct attack on the other sex. Males convicted of this offence show varying degrees of immaturity, are not outwardly aggressive, have a feeling of sexual inadequacy and carry out their offences in fleeting moments of impulse.

Young male adolescents with immature sex drives may make suggestions to children, undress them, spank them, simply look at them, and occasionally attempt to fondle their genital areas. One inmate I knew, an eighteen-year-old, was charged several times in one year for detaining little girls in a ravine, partially undressing them and spanking them. One conviction put him in reformatory for eight months and a second sent him to penitentiary as a dangerous sex offender. After eight years, he returned to society matured and stabilized. He got married and is now functioning well as an adult.

Indecent assault has many variations. It can be non-violent as in the case of the *huggers* and *feelers*, who get their jollies in the office, at parties and in crowds generally. Career women frequently are subjected to this kind of indignity. The "feel" is usually directed to one area of a woman's body. We refer to the act as a "dry rub," or to use the proper French word from which the English term is derived, "frottage."

People convicted of indecent assault involving a serious degree of violence usually end up in prison. Their personalities are poorly stabilized. They attempt to hide in the population, have few friends and are always in some kind of danger because of their actions on the street.

Incest involves sexual relations with relatives and a person convicted of it seldom has a repeat offence. I have seen at least a dozen cases, and the people involved, with sentences of less than five years, have all had stable backgrounds. One of my typical cases would involve a man of forty to fifty years of age with four to seven daughters. His wife is an overweight, poorly disciplined person with no interest in herself. To support the family, the husband has a regular job, a second job doing house repairs, and usually a third job selling wares in the community.

He develops fatigue from overwork, loses interest in his wife, resorts to alcohol and only then makes a sexual overture to one of his younger daughters. He chooses her as a sexual substitute for his wife and, in his fantasy, affronts his wife with the knowledge that he would rather have a relationship with his daughter than with her. Eventually, the relationship is disclosed, charges are laid, by the police or by the wife, and the father goes off to prison. It is paradoxical that the victimized daughter usually corresponds faithfully with the man during his incarceration.

In prison, men sentenced for incest are hard-working, industrious, quiet and very much aware of their folly. Interestingly enough, too, I have never known one of these inmates to be the subject of threats or injury from other prisoners.

The most dangerous of the sex offenders, insofar as children are concerned, are the pedophiles. They are not interested in adults, directing their aggression rather toward children, practicing everything from exhibitionism to sadistic acts which all too frequently end in murder. If the offender is a heterosexual male, his victim will be a young girl; and if he is homosexual, the victim will be a boy.

These offenders have a stormy time in prison. They are described as kid *diddlers* and are shunned and degraded at every turn. The pedophiliac who has a truly horrendous crime on his record usually does not live long in a penitentiary. He is murdered by a chosen inmate – and there are no witnesses and no convicting evidence.

Since they only like children, these inmates see no sexual activity behind bars. They perpetuate their fantasies, however. One man spent his time pasting birth notices of Toronto girls in his scrapbook. He had over three thousand entries over a four-year period.

Pedophiliacs choose their children from different age groups. Clinically, I have found that the preferred age of the victim parallels the age of the offender at a point in childhood when he had a significantly warm relationship with someone. For example, one inmate, reviewing his early history, remarked, "When I was eleven, my sister and I slept together every night when my parents were out drinking with their friends. She was ten and I always cuddled up to her. We felt we needed each other." This man's later life was a psychological tragedy. Never able to find the love and warmth he had known with his sister, he went looking for a substitute. He found it among ten-year-old girls.

There are many hidden sexual offenders among inmates doing time for such crimes as assault, wounding and unlawfully entering a house. That is to say, their crimes have a strong sexual connotation. It is estimated, incidentally, that ten per cent of all aggressive offences by males have a significant sexual component.

Dennis, twenty-three, was one of those hidden offenders. In 1976 he was sentenced to eight years imprisonment on no fewer than twenty-four charges of break and entry. In each case, he broke into a woman's apartment.

Dennis acted like a typical burglar. He would break into an apartment in the early hours of the morning and prowl about, picking up whatever took his fancy. But then the sexual element would take over. Instead of leaving, he would go into the bedroom and sit on the bed of the sleeping woman. If she did not awaken on her own, he would prod her until she did. He would remain then there until she opened her eyes and faced him, usually screaming. Moments later he would get up and slip quietly out of the apartment. He never harmed the women.

## CHAPTER 19

# An Experiment in Sensory Deprivation

I have to say I really like this old world of mine, aglow with its myriad of colors, alive with its countless precious sounds. Cumulus formations in the sky. Chopin on FM, the sun and rain on my face, the laughter of children in my home, the smell of Jane's potatoes baking in their jackets, the wonderfully-animated conversation that always occupies us all after dessert.

These are some of the sensory pleasures of my life. You, I am sure, have your own special variety. But what would life be like without these sensations? What would we be like if there were no color in our lives, no range of sound, no meaningful communication, no affection, none of the gratifications of physical and emotional experience?

We would be dull, unimaginative, uninspired robots. We'd be near-vegetables. We'd be victims of sensory deprivation.

This is a condition based on my theory of input-output. A man who receives a good deal of stimulation from his world is far more likely to be bright and interesting than one who locks it out.

It's not really unlike computer philosophy. What you program in, you can program out. Or as one jokester used to say, "Garbage in, garbage out."

The old adage that all work and no play makes Jack a dull boy had considerable currency at one time, but I somehow suspect that Jack's problem revolved around his lack of sensory input, aggravated, no doubt, by his job. If, in a nutritional sense, man is what he eats, then I think we'd have to say that, in a physical and emotional context, he has to be a reflection of what he absorbs.

My interest in sensory deprivation goes back to the early 1960's when I began observing a group of twenty-two particularly dull, lethargic inmates at Kingston Penitentiary. Some of them spent their days carrying mops and brooms around. Others worked in the vegetable gardens and on the grounds, raked the gravel, painted the stone walls, washed the windows. Most of them belonged to what we call the ornamental gang, that is they looked after the land and floral areas inside the walls.

What intrigued me about these twenty-two men was the fact that they were all long-termers and yet I knew none of them. As prison psychiatrist, I thought I knew all the oldtimers. Obviously, I didn't.

I checked with Jack Burke, the World War II veteran who ran our psychiatric unit at the time (he died in May 1981) and John Allen, the work supervisor in the trades office. The men, I discovered, were all lifers or were serving terms of many years.

"Bad criminals – but good inmates."

That's how John Allen described them. By good inmates, of course, he meant inmates who caused no trouble.

There was Jody who had murdered his wife and two children; Dutch who had staged a bank robbery; Bob, an habitual criminal – and a wide-ranging variety of miscreants.

What they seemed to have in common was a detachment from the world. Certainly on my input-output scale, they rated very low. They all liked working alone. They seldom spoke to one another. They never associated with other inmates. They never appeared on sick parade and never requested psychiatric interviews.

They were drab and virtually lifeless. They were there – that was all.

One night, while I was reading the paper at home, my son Michael came to me for help with a history essay he was writing about the trip to England of the famous French adventurers (and founders of the original Hudson's Bay Company) Raddison and des Grosseillers in the early 1700's.

"I call them Radishes and Gooseberries," Michael said. He paused, "Radishes are red, aren't they?"

I nodded.

"Well, what's red like? I don't know what red is." He paused again. "I don't know what green looks like. Or yellow. Or blue."

Of course, he couldn't recognize colors. He suffered from complete color blindness. He lived in a gray world.

Michael was an overactive boy. He was restless in class with a tendency to rise to answer all questions. He was also very talkative and at home he always kept his radio on extra loud.

I wondered if Michael was compensating for his lack of color resources by talking so much and insisting on high-volume music.

And my drab inmates? Could they be existing in a colorless environment? Were they suffering from some form of color blindness too?

Michael was fascinated by physical endurance. He'd cycle, swim and sometimes run until he was exhausted.

Could it be that people had to have sensation going into their bodies to keep them alert and interested? If so, had my lethargic prisoners exhausted all means of sensation and had they just given in to fatigue and boredom?

My curiosity was aroused.

I discussed my observations with the aunt of a boy with congenital blindness. She said her nephew had been an alarmingly restless child who frequently struck at the furniture with his fists in anger. A doctor friend of mine, with a mute child, told me about that boy's tendency to get angry and blow up.

"Sometimes," my friend explained, "he roams around the house like someone in a cage."

The next few nights, I sat in the medical library at Queen's University, making notes on boredom and its technical name, sensory restriction.

I read about children. Dr. George Kerr reported in the Journal of Pediatrics that youngsters reared without closeness and warmth failed to grow even though adequately nourished.

Without closeness and warmth. How many prisoners had grown up in such environments?

I read Dr. C. S. Mullins' report on the effects of boredom and isolation in five weather stations in Antarctica in the Journal of Psychiatry. It reinforced my original thinking.

For about six weeks, the report said, the stress of isolation caused restlessness, sleeplessness and a feeling of pent-up tension. After this period, the men lost interest in what they were doing, displayed a lack of intellectual energy, and a disinclination to study, write letters, or even work. Everyone seemed to become lethargic and mildly depressed. Animation was restored as the date approached for their return home.

The report reflected certain similar observations I had made in prison, especially concerning lethargy and lack of stimulation.

On a bright May morning in 1967, I decided to try something. I'm a person who loves color in everything and I had bought myself a red suit. Yes, red. A complete suit in red. This morning, then, I decided to go to work wearing it.

Jane laughed across the breakfast table, "You're going to work like that?" she asked.

"Yes," I answered. "This is my red day." I also had a green suit hanging in the closet and planned to wear it another day.

Shortly afterwards I passed through the two barred gates into the three-quarter acre rectangle of Kingston Penitentiary and ran into some of the lethargic inmates I was talking about.

"God, Doc," one of them said, giving me the once-over, "you the new fire chief?"

"Hey, Doc, is the joint on fire?" another asked, a big grin creasing his face.

My red suit had had its effect. A few yards of colored material and there was new animation in the old fortress. Yet, could it really be true that these passive men could be activated in such a simple way? I decided to do some further exploration by talking to some of them. What was it that they really missed most in prison?

Jody missed family life, the confusion of things at home, the noise of the children, the barking of the dog. Things like that.

Dutch missed women, booze and cars. "This place is like a human junkyard," he said. "Everyone is worn down, burned out or buggered up."

Warren, who had killed a bank messenger, missed the view of the countryside from his living room window. "I had a big picture window which looked west," he recalled. "What I saw there was a big part of my life."

In the psychiatric unit, I made brief notes. Jody had suffered a loss of family relationships; Dutch had lost his social relationships; Warren longed for his natural surroundings.

But one summary observation stood out in my notes: "The inmates on the work assignment in the quandrangle noticed the man in the red suit. It seemed to have an alerting effect upon their minds."

By February 1968, I had developed a theory which rightly or wrongly put my thinking into a logical order.

Animal life is preceded by plant life which eventually becomes endowed with a system of mobility to search out food and energy sources. Man is a biological plant with highly developed mobility characteristics. The skin of an animal, like the surface of a plant, has energy-converting properties and is the centre of life with skin and hair follicles, the eyes and the ears being special adaptations of the skin figment. The energizing effect of stimulation of visual, auditory and tactile senses spark the electrical or kinetic forces of the body.

The host of these processes is caloric man, a sophisticated version of the simple organic cell. Caloric man feeds on ingested plants and animals to produce carbohydrate energy required for various movements, including speech.

Cooking and heating of these plants and animals add both heat and caloric support for all body functions.

To summarize, man obtains his vital energy through his senses which supply the bio-electric circuits of the body, the brain, the heart, the skin. In effect, the electricity recorded on the electroencephalograph, the electrocardiograph and the galvanic skin currents must come from sensory input through skin and allied organs. Eating is a simple process of supplying foods of different qualities to the organic needs of man.

In terms of incarceration, I reasoned, a prisoner exists in a deprived state with a great monotony of light, sound, movement and color. Thus he has less kinetic energy to utilize his system effectively. The results are slow movement, fewer interests, lethargy, inability to concentrate and formulate plans and a lack of animation and sparkle in conversation.

Imprisonment is a type of social isolation in which there are few changes in the environment, limited variation in daily activities and minimal relationship and contact with the outside world. The mood and movements of the prison are slow, methodical, obsessive and unchanging.

The psychological flat lands are shadowed on all sides by thick grey walls, long grey corridors and guarded ranges with barred doors that look in upon blue-grey cells in which each bed is covered by a grey blanket. (Color only recently has existed in penal institutions and then in muted tones of yellow and green.)

Institutionalization is a condition where the individual is controlled by his environment in an obedient robot-like fashion. Institutional man does not appear suddenly. He is the product of slow transformation from an average youth with interests, ambitions and objectives into a quiet-moving, accepting person who lives in his environment without any feeling of personal rebellion or any awareness of the outside world.

Institutionalization affects a broad range of people. It is paradoxical that some persons prefer to withdraw into an inactive environment even though there are opportunities to function in response to others.

In the early years of the century, mental patients suffered from inertia, passivity and disinterest. Efforts to organize them into sports and trade interests, however, gave them new interests.

How I remember my early years as an intern in the Brockville Psychiatric Hospital, watching dull, grey men walk up and down the corridors shoving heavy brushes with the slow, laboring expression of weary oxen.

Social isolation is experienced by a formidable percentage of our population and includes such physical captives as the hemiplegic, the osteoarthritic, the aged, and mental patients who exist in the endless monotony of chronic wards.

I had delved deeply into institutionalization and theorized that each person required a basic amount of perceptual input a day. I believed man could produce this level through the perceptual feeling of his physical movements, through the perceptual sound of his own voice, and through an awareness of his own thoughts, all of which, I calculated, should produce restless and random activities. I developed the "need theory of optional sensory input" by which a person who hadn't much going for him in his life, would compensate by seeking other sense means to keep his interests active, much as a blind person develops hypersensitive hearing.

I had observed that color-blind boys were physically overactive, as was the case with Michael. I was also aware of something else – that a person who is ill for an extended period of time loses awareness of the passing days, becomes interested only in his personal life and functions, and accepts passivity as a way of life. In effect, boredom generates boredom. A drop in input from environment results in mental sluggishness: a disinclination in the area of effort, planning and motivation.

I discussed with three experienced psychologists, Doctor Nelson Freedman and Doctor J. G. Wilde of Queen's University, and Doctor Paul Gendreau, a senior psychologist who worked with me at Kingston Pentitentiary, the possibility of a research project involving inmates.

The question I wanted answered was this: Did complete sensory isolation produce any change in man's psychology and mental functions?

The project won the approval of Allen J. MacLeod, Q.C., who was then Commissioner of Penitentiaries. MacLeod, who probably did more to change the face of the old fortress prison mentality than anyone up until his time, was always intrigued with new ideas. In fact, many of the innovative ideas he developed in the 1960's are part of today's regular prison programs.

I won't labor the intricacies of research equipment. Seven inmates volunteered to engage in a program of complete sensory deprivation for a period of seven days, during which time they were housed in a dark sound-proof cell with limited movement. Radio telemetry recorded their physical movements. It was, in effect, a process of monitoring human functions by transmittor. (A second group of seven inmates acted as a control, spending seven days in a standard cell where they experienced normal institutional sound stimuli.)

The results were reported in the Journal of the Canadian Psychiatric Association. The conclusion reached was that there was a significant reduction in basic brain rhythm waves producing clinical changes of passivity and disinterest. Doctor Lorne Carpenter, senior psychiatric clinician at K.P., spoke to the inmates about their experiences.

Max stated that the most disturbing effect of being in the darkened cell was the darkness itself. After a time the room lost its dimensions, so that it seemed to him to be a round hall. He daydreamed, and stared for long periods at a pinhole of light over the window. He became fearful after the fourth day, the fear approaching panic level. He observed that sounds were much more acute when he returned to a normal environment but within a few hours his hearing adjusted.

Burt said that nothing disturbed him in the darkened cell. He said he could have gone on much longer. The darkness did not bother him and there was no time distortion. He knew when it was night and slept through it. Upon release he also observed that his hearing had grown more acute, becoming normal in a few hours.

Luc thought the environment would be harmful if the period of confinement was extended. He suggested that, after three or four months, an inmate would start to decline mentally and physically. It would appear that Luc did not suffer any subjective "reactive reactions" from his period of deprivation.

Theo said the most disturbing aspect of the experience was the monotony. Being without tobacco bothered him for the first two days. He hallucinated during the last two days. He believed he saw the face of his brother, who had died in 1962, in the blackened window. It appeared very real. After shaking his head and looking again, it vanished. He also believed he saw spiders on one occasion. The blackness of the room caused a distortion in dimension and, at times, there appeared to be no ceiling. He was unable to keep track of time accurately. Upon release, light and noises seemed accentuated but returned to normal within a few hours.

Drew went over the many events of his life. He commented that, looking back, he could see that a lot of things he had done were stupid. Under other circumstances he would not have bothered to reminisce or recall. Prior to the time of release, he became very restless and continued to recount the number of days that he had been in there. The last half hour seemed endless.

Harvey stated that the period in the deprivation cell had little or no effect upon him. He felt he had good control over himself and developed a routine of exercise to avoid boredom. There was no time distortion. Upon release, it seemed the light was very bright, but this was adjusted in a matter of a few hours. He recalled he concentrated on the most minute sound while in the cell and upon release talked too loudly. He was told by other persons that he was shouting, when he believed he was talking at normal volume.

Arnie said that within two hours of being in the dark he was unable to tell what time it was. This distortion was most marked during the first four days. He experienced difficulty in sleeping the last few nights. Arnie stated that he naturally wanted out as he was an energetic person. However, knowing ahead how long he had to remain in the cell was helpful. He kept track of the number of days on the wall.

Marvin said the darkness did not bother him. The thing that troubled him the most was the removal of his tobacco. He stated that the first few days were the most difficult. He was certain he could have gone another seven days.

The comments were interesting, but a Queen's University computerman's analysis of biochemical changes during the enforced isolation provided some indisputable hard-core facts.

The analysis showed a definite reduction in certain brain wave components from ten to eight cycles per second and indicated that a decline in certain brain waves co-related with apathetic, resigned behavior in subjects in the research module. It was also shown that, up to a seven day period, the brain wave decline was reversible.

Our research explained the psychiatric situation in prisons – fogging, coasting, the jitters. It also explained why the institutionalized inmate, living in a deprived setting, cannot adjust to a sudden release into free society. His mental and emotional mechanisms, are adjusted to chronic, deprived circumstances.

One of the important conclusions of the project was that adequate sensory stimulation must be introduced into maximum security centres to prevent the deprivation syndrome of disinterest and withdrawal.

We recommended increased use of piped-in radio to each cell, the installation of more television sets, more stimulating color schemes in the prison environment, and an increase in group meeting programs. We pointed out that an activity program to ensure adequate stimulation must also enthusiastically embrace the fields of education, shop training, trades instruction and a full-fledged physical exercise program.

I'm not sure that my kinetic theory impressed anyone. Our isolation project, however, was something else. I think I would be flattering myself and my associates by accepting the credit for what was accomplished. However, a great many changes took place in penitentiaries across Canada very soon after our work was completed. There was a definite awakening, a new awareness, that human automation could be changed through different prison activities.

It doesn't really matter where the stimulation comes from – as long as it's there. And it can come from seemingly insignificant things. Stimulation comes from having a good talk, or a good laugh, with someone. It can come from standing under a shower that has been adjusted for finer spray and increased pressure. It can come from punching a bag, and riding a bicycle. Sometimes, it can even come from seeing somebody walking into a dull, drab area wearing a red suit.

## CHAPTER 20

# Crime Denial and Confession

Psychiatry is not an exact science. Man's mind has many recesses. Behavior reflects the physical outcrop of the emotional and mental complexes within each separate personality. In crime, there are two strange phenomena: one of crime denial, the other of false confession, both of which, from time to time, obscure the true and predictable motivations basic to any criminal act.

Crime denial is an uncommon occurrence in criminal cases. Such denial, however, no matter the reason, leaves in its wake an uneasy feeling that the conviction may have been unjust. Many a judge and many a lawyer have uttered the old adage that it's better to free one hundred guilty men than to convict one innocent one. This is what underscores one of our basic legal concepts – that an accused man can be convicted only if his guilt has been proven beyond a reasonable doubt.

Criminal systems in the western world have such multiple safeguards built into them, that an act of injustice should never happen to an accused. We are speaking of the ideal, of course, because we know that injustice, though perhaps rare, is not unknown in the courts.

The simplest type of crime denial is that of "stubborn entrenchment", which is based on the belief that any statement an accused may make about himself can be used against him, and that any admission of fact concerning a criminal act is extremely dangerous.

This unrelenting denial is found in people who, themselves, are rigid and fearful of the consequences of any unwise act. For example, a boy may deny stealing a bicycle because he is fearful of his father's discipline. Denial may then become a part of his mentality, to the extent that he may refuse to give explanations for any of his acts. It occurs, too, in the very young, as in the case of a small boy who, with his hand in the cookie jar, denies that he is taking the biscuits. A child who is fearful of physical retaliation for even minor causes learns to deny wrongdoing in the hope that he may escape another beating.

Roger was fifty-two and had served four years of a ten-year life sentence for murdering his wife when I saw him. He was an intolerant, argumentative person, best described as an angry loud-mouth. In his own community he fought with his neighbors, hassled the township council and had no friends. He had been convicted on a mass of solid circumstantial evidence, though his wife's body had never been found.

In consultations with me concerning his difficulties in adjusting to prison, he frequently mentioned his conviction but always denied killing his wife. He had organized his mind into rigid compartments, which he could open or close off at will. He showed no feelings about his wife's death, only anger at his conviction. During all of our sessions, he acted as though he honestly believed he was innocent.

I gave a good deal of thought to Roger's case and it was my belief that he had knowingly refused to save his wife's life in a crucial set of circumstances. He had pushed her from a boat in deep water and then hurried across the bay to get help to rescue her. He may not, in effect, have killed his wife. He may simply have placed her in a situation which resulted in her death.

Stubborn entrenchment is frequently seen in childhood and adolescence where the subject immediately denies any wrongdoing and does not alter his attitude because there would be too many necessary explanations.

Then there is occasional denial, where the accused temporarily will deny the crime because of possible physical harm. Not long ago a youth of eighteen was accused of killing a fifty-seven-year-old railroad worker. He was so insistent that he was innocent, that his lawyer had me look into the case. I suggested he be moved to a jail in my area. Transferred there, he settled in and within two days had written me a reasonable story of his part in the murder. He stated he was fearful of being mistreated by the local police force because he had given them good cause to dislike him before this particular offence.

Crime denial may also involve the psychological defence mechanism of repressing the memory of a traumatic event. This may happen when an individual is exposed to some catastrophic incident which is overwhelming to his emotions and to his mind.

Psychiatrists see this mechanism frequently. I recall such a repressive amnesia in a fifty-eight-year-old woman. I was visiting her and her husband. He left the room to answer the telephone, suffered a massive coronary attack and was dead in five minutes. The wife stood near as I examined him. I told her to sit in the living room while I called the family doctor. When I re-entered the living room she said, "Alf has gone downtown and should be back in half an hour." It was forty-eight hours before her emotions let the tragic incident through to her conscious mind. This type of repressive amnesia is usually found in tense, compulsive, over-controlled people who do not easily show their true emotional selves. Crying and anger are infrequently expressed.

The young and teenage personality do not have this mechanism unless the individual has a long history of emotional maladjustments in terms of physical complaints with vague symptoms, and a tendency to be preoccupied with his own interests.

Crime denial may have its basis in the actual mental processes of a person. Such individuals symbolically have two minds. One is functional in terms of reality and the other is totally given to highly-involved fantasies, usually of an angry nature. These frequently have their beginnings in hurtful relationships with a father, mother, brother or sister. It then becomes extended to individuals who have the habits and mannerisms of hated family members.

The person manages to cling to reality unless some traumatic incident, usually of a frustrating nature, awakens his fantasy and sparks a course of violent action, a retaliation against some hurtful figure of the past carried out on some innocent hapless person.

In children and adolescents, the individual is usually identified as a seclusive person who does not encourage close relationships. These young people resemble the schizophrenic-reaction type with marked emotional apathy, a serious level of controlled anger, and a vivid, mind-occupying, hostile fantasy life.

At an earlier period, the person may realize that the other mind is interfering with his everyday life and its adjustments. If some trigger mechanism explodes the anger, the person may actually feel he did nothing wrong and that it was the sick part of his mind that made him do the act. The person may believe he did no harm, that Z4 did the harmful thing. There may be, in serious cases, a loss of personal identity and a substitution of a deceitful personality which commands behavior from time to time.

Another type of denial is based on the conviction that there was no unlawful act, that the person was wrongly accused and that the evidence had been misleading and incorrect. In effect, the arrest, trial and conviction had been a complete miscarriage of the legal process.

There is also an outside runner in crime denial. He is not in the same category as the simple-denial people. He races under the name of automatism. In this condition, there is a temporary loss of the conscious mind, although the body is still able to move freely, combined with automatic or involuntary action. The picture of a stunned boxer staggering around the ring in a boxing stance is a simple example of the state of automatism. In effect, the boxer does not know what he is doing or what he intends to do. If, for instance, he returned to the dressing room in his dazed state and killed his manager by a blow to the head, without any conscious intent, it could be reasoned he was not guilty of killing him.

To cite another example, a teenager might take a dose of LSD or ingest six ounces of whisky. If he were unfamiliar with the effects of the drug, or the alchohol, he might commit acts which he would not remember. The courts could then consider his case on the basis of automatism, which could well exonerate him from responsibility for the offence.

In all cases, however, my old rule stands: the crime has to fit the personality of the offender.

For instance, robberies and assaults are carried out by aggressive people, fraud by somewhat controlled, well-educated and very manipulative persons. Thieves are usually devious, non-productive and poorly-educated. Sex offenders have impoverished emotional development and gain perverse, emotional satisfaction from their offences.

People who combine crimes of assault, robbery, forgery, car theft and indecent assault have no specific criminal pattern. These multiple characteristics however, indicate they are mentally ill.

The personality rule, however, raises serious doubts in certain cases. I am thinking of a boy I'll call Jeff. Jeff was convicted of sex murder of a nine-year-old girl named Lynn in Peterborough in 1971. He was sixteen at the time. He appealed, was granted a new trial and was convicted a second time.

Jeff has maintained his innocence steadfastly ever since his arrest. I have seen him a number of times at Beaver Creek Institution, where he is serving a life sentence, and he adamantly denies that he committed the crime. I have assessed him over the years and have come to the conclusion that he doesn't have the personality of a murderer.

There are a number of similarities between Jeff's story and the more celebrated case of Steven Truscott some twelve years earlier. To begin with, all of the players in these two tragedies were children. Steven, at fourteen, was two years younger than Jeff when convicted of raping and killing Lynne Harper (Lynne with an e in this case). She was twelve. Both boys vehemently denied responsibility for the murders. Both were convicted on circumstantial evidence.

Jeff's case never generated the great national interest stirred by the Truscott affair. I suspect, however, that one of the reasons for this is that no one thought to write a book about young Jeff. (Three were written about Truscott).

**Confessions**

The undetected crime is not a technical crime. It is an event which passes below the conscious level of social man as a criminal act. The act itself is carried out by a human being and, to be a crime, it has to be discovered by another human being.

The percentage of unsolved crimes is believed to be much higher than that of solved crimes. There is little difference between the criminal and the non-criminal man, just a matter of detection and conviction. Isolated criminal acts happen with great frequency, but many minor ones are too insignificant to prosecute.

The word confession has mixed emotional tones, but may be described as an oral or written acknowledgement of guilt by a party accused of an offence. Criminal man looks upon a confession with great contempt, with the view that guilt for any crime has to be proven. Why help the prosecution?

Confessions, admissions, statements and declarations have a legal oneness and may be inculpatory (incriminating) or exculpatory (clear of guilt). Statements have to be made freely and voluntarily. They cannot be raised in court unless the presiding judge says they are admissible. The rules are strict. A confession which is prompted by fear of prejudice, or hope for advantage, is not considered true. Also, when confessions are received by persons other than policemen, it becomes a matter of vital importance whether such persons possessed actual authority.

For instance, a recent confession, made in jail by an accused to a policeman posing as a criminal, was considered valid. Even crime informants, prosecution witnesses and victims of crime are considered to have authority in most cases.

A surgeon, called to a jail, told an accused he had better "tell all". In this case, however, the ensuing evidence was not admissible. Even veiled reference to a guilty act can be made inadmissible if given to a doctor.

Psychiatrists find themselves, from time to time, examining an accused person or prison inmate and obtaining information relevant to his crime, or to other crimes. A psychiatrist in private is not considered a person in authority, but a prison psychiatrist functions in an environment of authority, hence his information is not admissible in a court of law. The presiding judge usually considers the statements of the private psychiatrist admissible.

As in other areas of our justice system, there are safeguards for the accused. If an accused is in custody for an offence, a statement about another offence is non-admissible. Any offer to the accused such as promise of bail, of psychiatric help or "off the record" help, negate the validity of any admission.

One type, however, is admissible in court. That is the volunteered confession.

Some marginally mentally ill people have a strong need to confess to a crime, based upon exaggerated feelings of unworthiness.

In a penitentiary, troubled inmates may seek help of the psychiatrist and in the process disclose information about certain criminal acts. For example, someone might say, "I've made my living by fraud. Mostly cheques. I am rather well off. I expect to be caught from time to time but it's a game with me."

Other inmates involved in break and entry charges may indicate that they have lived on the income from stolen goods, and may even relate a number of their illegal adventures.

Admissions of serious offences are uncommon, but may be made in such detail that the stories appear authentic. One case in 1974 involved Ian, a thirty-year-old man who was admitted to the psychiatric unit at Kingston Penitentiary in a state of agitation and depression. He saw me at weekly intervals with confessions of four different crimes involving attacks on young girls, mature women and aged ladies. Each case was presented with an accompanying description, complete with house layouts, highway numbers, proximity to various cities and other details. I could detect obvious signs of longstanding aggressive fantasies towards all women.

In appearance, Ian was a short-statured man with a drawn, expressionless face and a very passive, colorless voice. He walked with a stoop and had an ominous presence.

His confessions increased and I advised him that I was in no position to act on his information. If he wished, however, I could obtain a lawyer who would give him substantial advice concerning his disclosures.

He seemed to withdraw from this suggestion. It was obvious to me that he was not convinced that he really had been responsible for all these offences. As his mental depression increased, I arranged, with his permission, to send him to the Mental Health Centre, Penetang, for evaluation and treatment.

I completed my referral information and enclosed copies of his drawings and directions. One particular drawing of an apartment layout seemed so detailed that I asked him to do a second drawing on the pretext that I had lost the original. Again he drew from memory producing a sketch of the same apartment, same size living room, bedroom, kitchen and bathroom, complete with location of the stove and refrigerator.

I watched as he used an eraser several times to place chairs and tables in their proper position. He then remarked "Here I sat with Maggie. I raped her on the floor then I buggered her over the table. I dressed her, ran the water in the bath tub and drowned her. I took all the money I could find."

I considered that perhaps Ian had an ongoing adolescent-like fantasy based on some story he had read in a detective magazine. But on the possibility of it being true fact, I communicated with the Homicide Division of the Toronto Metropolitan Police. A sergeant-detective named Detler telephoned back in two days with no evidence that Maggie so-and-so had been murdered. The police had absolutely no record of her death.

The Mental Health Centre also reviewed my information about Maggie and believed it to be sexual rumination. After a year at Penetang, my patient was transferred to a hospital in his home area. Here he remained through the winter months, quiet and well-behaved. He was given walking privileges on several occasions.

In jail in Brockville, Ian spoke again of Maggie. This time Sergeant-Detective Detler and a fellow officer from Toronto homicide visited him. Ian again reviewed Maggie's death. The detective returned to Toronto to find no record of an unsolved homicide. By this time both detectives were at a loss. Then one decided to review the obituary notices in the Toronto papers for the dates mentioned by Ian. And there it was – an obituary notice for Maggie. Detectives then visited her next-of-kin, who had assumed that she had fallen into the bathtub and drowned. Checking with her brother, police discovered that Ian had drawn an accurate sketch of the apartment.

Ian was transferred to jail in Toronto and charged formally with the murder of Maggie. He became suspicious and apprehensive and, at the preliminary hearing, was declared unfit to stand trial because of a mental condition that made him incapable of understanding his situation. Four months later, he faced trial and was declared legally insane.

Ian's background was as traumatic and horrible as his offences. He was the only child of a single, mentally retarded, alcoholic mother who beat him frequently. Police said he was in and out of court on countless occasions. They described his early life as appalling, recalling how he caught pigeons in the coal lofts and pulled their wings apart.

Ian's confession to me was more of a self-flattering review of his sexual achievement and domination over Maggie in the last few hours of her life. He recalled his orgy of destruction over and over, and from it obtained a feeling of fulfillment. Each drawing of the apartment stirred him sexually, which satisfied his anger and resentment toward his depraved and vicious mother. Truly a very sick and ruthless person.

Ian is now slumbering away within the safe confines of the Mental Health Centre, Penetang.

## CHAPTER 21

# Steven Truseott: A Personal Investigation

I don't know whether my late friend, Victor Richmond, regional director of penitentiaries for Ontario, was paying me a compliment, or reminding me that I was becoming a nuisance, but I like to think that he came pretty close to the truth when he said, "Scott, you're a hell of a guy once you get something in your head."

Well, I did have something in my head and it was bugging me.

It was Steven Truscott.

In the realm of crime denial, the Truscott case has to be a classic. It is the story of a man who has been proclaiming his innocence for nearly a quarter of a century and who, in the eyes of the law, remains a convicted murderer.

It has always been assumed among penitentiary officials that people who are behind bars are there because they are guilty. It is, of course, not an illogical assumption since very few innocent individuals actually wind up in jail.

But I'm not strong on assumptions. I look for reasons, and for explanations. And when the pieces don't fit the puzzle, it bothers me.

"Scott's playing detective," someone scoffed one day, implying, I think, that I was a psychiatrist and should confine my talents to that particular profession.

Before I was through, however, I had enlisted the support of a number of people in my investigations – not only penitentiary officials but Justice Department representatives as well. And I had involved myself in activities far removed from the psychiatric couch.

But let's go back to the beginning.

Steven Murray Truscott was the son of Warrant Officer Dan Truscott and his wife Doris, and lived on the former Royal Canadian Air Force station at Clinton, Ontario. In June of 1959, at age fourteen, he was arrested and charged with the rape and murder of Lynne Harper, twelve-year-old daughter of Flying Officer and Mrs. Leslie Harper, who also lived on the base.

In the fall of 1959, he was tried for murder, convicted and sentenced to be hanged. He spent four months in a death cell in the old jail at Goderich, expecting the hangman to put the noose about his neck. His death sentence finally was commuted to one of life and he was sent to the Ontario Training School at Guelph. At age eighteen, he was transferred into adult incarceration at Collins Bay Penitentiary.

The arrest and trial generated considerable sympathy for him. The sentence – death for a fourteen-year-old – swelled the feeling. In 1966, Toronto writer Isabel LeBourdais' "The Trial of Steven Truscott" created a great new swell of sympathy for him. Truscott, LeBourdais charged, had been tried improperly in an openly hostile court. The book led to a new hearing of the case by the Supreme Court of Canada. The majority report of the Supreme Court, in effect, upheld the ruling of the lower court and Steven's position remained unchanged.

I began seeing Steven in consultation in 1963, three years before the LeBourdais book made him one of the most talked-about individuals in the country. My interviews were to continue until he was released on parole.

I made the situation plain at the first consultation. There were three possibilities, I told him: one, that he was guilty of the murder of the girl; two, that he was protecting someone else who had committed the crime; and, three, that some unlikely coincidence had placed him squarely in the seat of guilt. He said the third explanation was correct.

I gathered psychiatric and psychological reports that had been prepared for the trial and others from the Guelph reformatory. I was digging into this individual's life, examining him, analyzing him. I wanted to understand his personality in the early years. I wanted to know him *now*.

Did he reveal evidence of explosive aggressiveness, temper tantrums or sleep disorders in his childhood development?

Did he show hostile aggressive characteristics in prison? Was there evidence of impulsivity and turbulence in the aggravating world of prison politics?

I explored the possibility of his having an "inner life," that is a fantasy life in which he dreamed of achieving certain goals, in which he expressed his anger and frustration in mind-role playing. If fantasies existed, there would be signs of preoccupation, lack of attention and difficulty in concentration.

I recalled the amnesia theory put forward by my longtime friend and advisor, the late neuro-psychiatrist, Dr. J. P. S. Cathcart. Truscott, he said, was guilty but was incapable of admitting it, perhaps even to himself, as his sense of guilt would be too overwhelming.

Was it possible that he had ingested some street drug such as LSD?

Could he have taken a large dose of alcohol? These might have robbed him of memory of ensuing events. From information gathered, I could rule out both suggestions.

I covered a good deal of ground during those first three years studying my patient. I had made an evaluation of his pre-offence personality and studied the effect on him of the overwhelming stress caused by his arrest, the emotional trauma of the trial and the almost incapacitating experience of having spent three years in a reformatory.

My psychiatric relationship with Steven soon became a matter of national interest and curiosity. The newspapers were full of half-truths, veiled allegations and folklorish misconceptions about psychiatric treatment techniques. Reporters even stopped me in the street to ask my opinion on the case.

What was really happening behind the closed doors of my office was that I was getting to know Steven Truscott. And I had come to some conclusions, some positive ones.

There was no stubborn entrenchment here. Steven wasn't worried that he would make a statement harmful to him.

It was definitely not a question of repressive amnesia. He didn't have any sense of guilt so great that he refused to recognize it.

There was no personality disorganization in his development as a youth. He had the average unexceptional history of academic, sports and social participation typical of the developing teenager.

After three years of interviews, I reworded my first statement to him. "Steven," I said, "there are three possibilities in a case of this kind. A person may be shielding someone near him; he might not wish to accept his own guilt; or he may just not know anything about the situation at all."

Steven, always cooperative, always polite, said nothing. He just looked at me – and I knew what he was thinking. He had said he was innocent so many times before.

I didn't need to say anything more. The crime has to fit the personality of the offender. It was my own basic philosophy.

Murder didn't fit the personality of Steven Truscott.

And that's when my detective work began in earnest.

"She had been frightfully mistreated. Someone had attempted to have sexual intercourse with her and had damaged her frightfully."

The words of Mr. Justice Ferguson at Steven's trial came back to me. I also recalled the evidence of a witness that an examination of Lynne's body indicated she may have been raped more than once. She may even have been the victim of a multiple rape.

The personality of the offender.

What kind of person would commit a crime like this? I went to bed that night thinking about it. I woke the next morning thinking about it.

I began conjecturing. Perhaps the real killer of Lynne Harper would end up in prison on some other charge. Perhaps it would be for a similar kind of offence. Then again, he might already be in prison.

I had already decided that this was not the crime of a schoolboy.

My history-taking of inmates always included their record of employment over the recent past. I dug deep into those records. Perhaps someone I interviewed would have been in the area of Clinton in June of 1959. "God, Scott," I mused out loud one day, "you sure like playing long shots."

Maybe I'm lucky. Maybe I live right. How else can I explain coming across an inmate who had been working as a painter in the general area of Clinton in June of 1959? He had come into Kingston Penitentiary in 1964 on a bank robbery conviction.

Could he be the killer? It was not impossible, I reasoned. But there was another possibility – his brother, who was also in K.P. I checked on the latter and discovered that he was a very rough individual with pronounced aggressive hostile characteristics. They had been painting light standards at service stations together in 1959, along with a third man, who was ex-inmate of K.P.

About this time, I was getting additional information from someone I regarded as a knowledgeable informant. My first suspect, he said, had been talking about a murder that had happened some years earlier. A little girl had been raped and killed and he was accusing his brother of doing the deed. Could he be talking about Lynne Harper? I was intrigued.

I gathered up my notes and went to see a warm, intelligent, professional colleague of mine. "You know," I said, "we might just be on to something here." Later we discussed the matter with Victor Richmond and got the go-ahead. We were to proceed with our investigation.

It was a most unusual situation, perhaps even unique. Here we were, two psychiatrists, following a kind of will-of-the-wisp, trying to find a new solution to a case that Justice, in all her wisdom, had declared solved years before. As for Steven Truscott, he was serving out his time at Collins Bay, entirely unaware of what we were doing.

I began my work by sifting through five volumes of Truscott trial evidence and notes on subsequent events, provided me by George Street, then Chairman of the National Parole Board. I wanted to be intimately familiar with every aspect of the case. I supplemented my reading by checking on newspaper accounts.

"I told him to confess, that it would be a lot easier for him if he did."

A Toronto paper quoted these words from an interview with Dr. J.

A. Addison, a Clinton doctor who examined Truscott shortly after the murder. The statement irked me. The man who was speaking was not a police officer but simply a general practitioner. And I said so.

Then came a reprimand. Prison psychiatrists, an official reminded me, have to assume that their inmate-patients are guilty of the crimes for which they have been convicted.

But I kept saying, over and over to myself, the crime must fit the personality of the offender.

I did the basic studies and laid the groundwork but my colleague did the leg work – and what a job he did. He did it all on his own time because there could be no formal authorization from the service. On weekends when he wasn't working, he visited the murder area, talked to dozens of people, made notes on all kinds of information he had picked up.

He even visited the parents and other relatives of the men I had seen in prison. What a gutsy guy, going into those homes and asking all kinds of personal questions concerning our subjects' backgrounds, their criminal activities, their potential for violence. I'm not at all sure I would have had the nerve to do what he did. My friend's interviews produced a good many facts, one of them being that at least one of the subjects had a tremendous potential for violence and was indeed capable of committing murder.

"You're a hell of a guy," I said when he returned from one of his expeditions.

He was quiet and just shrugged at my comment. Later, he told me he had been threatened. One of our subjects had warned him to quit bothering him, or face the consequences. Whatever they were.

But he doesn't bow to threats, so we went on with our work. From people in Seaforth, a town a few miles from Clinton, we learned that three men had been painting service station standards in the area at the time of the murder, working as employees of a Toronto construction firm.

We hired an investigator to check Toronto construction companies. One had contracted to paint in the Seaforth area. Our investigator checked the employment records and found the names of our two subjects at K.P. and their friend, who had been released. They had indeed been working in Seaforth on the night of the killing.

There was still another important link to be established. I had learned from my informant that the painters had travelled to Toronto soon after the time of the murder in a 1958 Ford station wagon and that they had abandoned the vehicle on a city street when it ran out of oil. Our investigator unfortunately could find no trace of that car.

I suppose some people would consider us amateurs in the investigation field but we spent more than three months building a file I called "The Case of the Three Painters." And we were convinced we were on the trail of important new evidence. Actually, certain penitentiary officials thought so too, since we got authorization to present a brief on our work to the Ontario Attorney-General's Department.

It was in September 1966 that we turned our brief with its bulging files over to the late W. C. Bowman, Director of Public Prosecutions. Later that month, he returned the documents with a note saying they had been photocopied. Two months later Bowman wrote to me again, this time to say that an inquiry was being made and that the Department of Justice was paying the costs.

My friend and I returned to our routine work and waited for news of the inquiry into our investigations. None came, and to this day there has been silence in officialdom.

Was the inquiry made? Did they check out our information? Did they investigate the painters?

Quite simply, we don't know.

I continued to see Steven Truscott at monthly intervals after this. (I never mentioned our work to him.) The interviews served to reaffirm my earlier assessment of him – that there were no dangerous elements in his personality.

In 1969, the question of Steven's parole came up. He had then served ten years of his life sentence and was eligible for parole consideration. However, there were problems. For one thing, his parents had separated. For another, he had little in the way of financial resources. Where would he go on release, and how could he look after himself financially?

I hoped to win unconditional freedom for Steven with my detective efforts but I had failed. Now I decided to try to help him in the normal process of parole. I called my present co-author, Bill Trent, then a staff writer for the nationally-circulated Weekend Magazine, and explained the circumstances. The wheels were turning full steam in my head. Steven needed to prove he had financial stability for release, and the writer, I knew, had been wanting to do his story for some time. The Parole Board, meantime, looked favorably on the plan.

Trent discussed the matter with the editors of Weekend Magazine and the response was both immediate and favorable. Yes, they wanted to publish the personal story of Steven Truscott. When finally Steven walked through the gates of Collins Bay Penitentiary on parole, it was with a contract from Weekend's parent firm, The Montreal Standard Publishing Company. That contract put a sizeable lump sum in Steven's bank account (particularly sizeable in terms of 1970 dollars,) thus assuring him of a good start on his re-entry into free society.

That, however, was not the end. The Montreal Standard, represented by Michael S. Baxendale, then negotiated a book deal with Simon & Schuster (Canada) Ltd. What emerged was "The Steven Truscott Story," a best-seller which dealt with Steven's life from the day of his arrest to his release on parole, and on which he earned royalties for years.

I cite this information as an example of what can be accomplished through cooperative effort. Certainly those of us in the Penitentiary Service and on the Parole Board who had been involved directly with Steven Truscott were gratified to know that he had been taken care of financially and that he would not be destitute once he reached the street.

It is worthy of mention, too, that over a period of several years following publication "The Steven Truscott Story," Bill Trent conducted a personal investigation into the case, checking out a multitude of claims and allegations from people who maintained that Steven was innocent. Some of these people went even further, claiming they knew the identity of the real killer, or killers.

My own enthusiasm for amateur detective work prompts me to applaud such individual effort. However, something more concrete than applause resulted here. Trent took his investigational reports to Michael Baxendale, now president of Optimum Publishing International, Inc., and suggested there was a book to be done. Baxendale, caught up in the implication of my report, decided to publish it in the hope that the real killer or killers might be found. The result was "Who Killed Lynne Harper?," a book that delved even further into the Truscott mystique.

Steven lives in a small town somewhere in Canada under an assumed name. He is married to a girl who petitioned for a Supreme Court hearing into his case back in the 60's. He is the father of three children and holds a responsible job in an industrial firm. Is he happy? I don't know. We are not in touch with one another. We said our goodbyes at Collins Bay.

Bill Trent's first book, "The Steven Truscott Story," won him a great many friends. His second book, "Who Killed Lynne Harper?," added to the list. It also sparked a new inquiry by the Attorney-General's Department. Nothing has come of that inquiry. It suffered the same fate as the inquiry into my own investigations. It died somewhere along the way. And so, in the eyes of the law, Steven Truscott remains the convicted murderer of Lynne Harper.

I still have a gut feeling, though, that someone else sleeps each night with the haunting memory of having killed that little girl.

**CHAPTER 22**

# Guards: Front-Line Story

Close relationships are a basic part of our personality structure. Man seeks friendships, enjoys being trusted and accepts the responsibilities of such situations. Then there is another kind of relationship we call "alien friendship." It is the condition that exists between prison guard and inmate.

Each functions in close contact with the other, watching the other and anticipating the other. In many cases, each is interdependent, one upon the other. Each meets frequently under a flag of tolerance, returning later to his lines to interpret the significance of recent conversations.

An inmate who crosses the psychological lines to communicate covertly with an officer is looked upon with suspicion. An officer who develops a more than passive interest in inmate matters finds himself openly ridiculed as a con-lover.

Much has been written about inmates, their problems, interests and human tragedies but little is really known about the men on the other side of the barrier and about the reactions that take place in this unique alien friendship.

Each prison function has guidelines specific for its purpose. There are directives for education, industrial training, maintenance, health care, supplies and services; in fact, for practically everything. But security forms the pyramid base upon which all of these departments depend.

On an average day, in an average institution, more than sixty per cent of the inmates are involved in some type of employment task. During the day, they move from one area to another, to carry out their duties, to keep medical appointments, meet visitors, go to the gymnasium, get their hair cut. Security has the responsibility of monitoring these movements, to ensure the safety of staff and inmates. Security has to be everywhere. There is even a program of preventive security which actually attempts to predict the likelihood of incident, serious and otherwise.

What kind of men perform security duties? Well, to begin with, there are no prima donnas among them. Experience is their teacher. There is no handbook, no educational degree, to give them special qualifications. You get to be chief keeper the hard way. The keepers are veterans of trouble. They know security is a bitter, thankless job – but they also know that a lack of incidents behind the walls is a tribute to their efforts.

I have seen an officer carrying an inmate dying of stab wounds in the chest down a long corridor and through several barriers to medical emergency, where waiting help rushed him to surgery.

I have seen officers move emotionally, from passive reserve into a very involved effort, to resuscitate an inmate after a serious suicidal event.

I have also been with officers as they waited for the coroner to remove the still warm body of a murder victim, killed swiftly by a single knife thrust through the heart.

Each officer is aware that he is less than two seconds away from a similar fate. In my own work, I depend on the security officer reaching me within seconds if I'm attacked. Great caution has to be taken interviewing new, unpredictable individuals, particularly mentally ill, delusional inmates.

You never know what's going to happen inside a penitentiary, but seasoned guards have always held to the belief that just about anything can happen. The point was proven on November 21, 1980 when the first armed robbery in Canadian prison history took place at Collins Bay Institution.

It was the biggest news event of the year behind the walls. It shocked the guards and shook the grapevine.

The inmate news hotline said it all in five words:

"They knocked off Disneyland today."

Two hooded inmates – the hoods were made from the leg of a suit of long underwear – walked into the vocational training office brandishing ten-inch knives, and ordered the duty officer to lie face down on the floor and his secretary to sit on a chair. They took $50 from the officer's wallet but got nothing from the secretary who had left her purse in another area. Ripping the telephone from the wall, they then slipped quickly and quietly out of the office.

Investigating officers hit the proverbial stone wall head-on when they began asking questions. Nobody had seen anything. Nobody had heard anything. Everybody was down with laryngitis again. The old-timers on the staff, of course, were hardly surprised.

What we're dealing with here is a brotherhood of danger.

Security officers are the defence corps of each institution. Personal discipline is self-imposed. Beginning with the inmate count in the morning, and going through noon and evening counts, the officers make it their duty to know the whereabouts of every inmate at all times.

Officers often are the target of well-meaning psychologists, sociologists and media people whose investigations and research studies have assessed many areas of their lives. Actually, officers' lives aren't all that different to those of merchants, tradesmen, or factory workers. The only truly remarkable difference is the danger element. The prison worker knows he is in a potentially dangerous environment. He knows that he himself may be injured, or even killed, and he is aware that the safety of his co-workers depends on his abilities. The risk variables are not insignificant.

Over the past twenty years, thirteen correctional officers, one of them a woman, have been killed. Eighty others have been wounded. And nearly five hundred have been involved in various hostage-taking incidents.

Guard William C. Wentworth, forty-two, was stabbed to death by one of twenty inmates occupying a dormitory at Kingston Penitentiary in November 1961. As usual, the inmates clammed up.

Officer Raymond J. Tellier, thirty-four, was stabbed fatally at St. Vincent de Paul Penitentiary in Québec in May 1963.

Classification Officer Mary Elizabeth Steinhauser, thirty-two, was shot in a hostage-taking incident at British Columbia Penitentiary in June 1975.

Officer Paul Gosselin, thirty-four, of Archambault Institution at Ste. Anne des Plaines, Québec, was stabbed while escorting an inmate to hospital, also in June of 1975.

Warden Michel Roy, thirty-nine, of Archambault Institution, was shot to death on the front lawn of his home by two ex-inmates in 1978.

The other officers murdered were:

Edwin James Masterton, Dorchester Penitentiary, Dorchester, N.B., died September 1964;

Georges Nadeau, forty-two, Cowansville Institution, Cowansville, Qué., died April 1975;

Roy William Eddy, forty-four, Regional Psychiatric Centre, Abbotsford, B.C., died in 1975;

Stanley Green, fifty-one, Stoney Mountain Penitentiary, Stoney Mountain, Manitoba, died 1974;

Francis Arthur Eustace, fifty-six, Collins Bay Penitentiary, Kingston, Ontario, died in November 1978;

Joseph Daniel Maurice, forty, Collins Bay Penitentiary, murdered in same incident as Francis Eustace;

Guy Fournier, twenty-nine, Laval Institution, Laval, Qué., died in July 1978;

William A. Morrison, forty-four, Dorchester Penitentiary, Dorchester, N.B., died October 1978.

There are no monuments to these people. They simply died in the performance of their dangerous duties. It's for this reason that I include them here – so that they won't be forgotten entirely

There is no major risk "position." Inmates who have killed guards have not displayed any obvious signs of being dangerous, or perhaps I should say of being more dangerous than others. When an officer is killed, it's because he is at a certain place at a certain time. Of course, there is little satisfaction in knowing that some guard was on the wrong shift at the wrong time.

Yet, there are degrees of apparent risk. I am thinking of the Special Handling Unit at Millhaven Institution which looks after about eighty of Canada's most dangerous criminals. So-called dangerous inmates are not that different from other prisoners, except that they can become really dangerous under certain aggravating conditions, such as home worries, resentments and mental delusions.

Truly dangerous men are rare. The most potentially explosive inmates are to be found in the twenty to thirty-year-old age group. As the years go by, the explosiveness tends to diminish.

One extremely dangerous inmate confided to me one day that he had done everything violent there was to do. His violent period, he said, came to an end in May 1979 when he slashed himself. "You know what, Doc," he explained, "I was lying there in my own blood, and for some reason or other, I said to myself, 'What the hell is all this stupidity about?' " As if by self-command, he changes his lifestyle. Today, he is reasonable, tolerant and hoping that one day he will be out of jail. He has three years to go before parole consideration.

I have spent much time relating to these special security inmates and to the officers of the Special Handling Unit and the work has been enlightening. Staff members are aware they are working in a dangerous zone here and each man knows his job is crucial to his colleagues. Interestingly enough, the men who handle Canada's toughest criminals are generally community-minded as well. More than thirty per cent of them, for example, are managing or coaching hockey, baseball and swim teams and helping young people in other ways.

There is no particular image of a correctional officer. He is an average man with a demanding job, reasonable pay and an adequate pension system. His employer will never go bankrupt and he can only lose his job through his own ineffectiveness. There are complainers and gripers among the custodial staffs, and activists too, who see imperfections in the system, as they would in any system. They are, however, rare. Also rare is the officer who uses his position to express his own aggression and hostility. Such men usually resign over the years because of inner tensions.

I have become aware of the problems of custodial recruits, having taught prison psychiatry to them for some fifteen years. Their eight-week courses cover security, inmate training, first aid, self-defence, weapons training, inmate discipline, emergency procedures together with thirty hours of psychiatric instruction. Recruits came from all walks of life – from merchant-class people to university graduates. During the last six years, however, a more highly-qualified group of recruits has been taken on strength. The group includes a sizeable complement of military men with at least ten years experience in the services. Military personnel accounted for twelve per cent of recruits in 1975, twenty-six per cent in 1978 and forty per cent in 1981. University degrees were held by nine per cent of recruits in 1975, twenty-two per cent in 1978 and fourteen per cent in 1981. Today's recruits are much more career-oriented than their predecessors.

Being a custodial person is not an easy job. I make that clear at the start. Officers are required to have the same qualifications as police recruits in terms of age, height, health and emotional stability. Unlike policemen, however, they have no weapons with which to defend themselves, while inmates have access to smuggled guns, home-made zip guns, stilettoes and knives, plastic or otherwise.

Time is the factor that modifies all behavior. It does so for inmates – and for the custodial officer. In the case of the latter, it can make damaging inroads that affect their attitudes and interests, and even their lives. One tends to think of prison syndromes as inmate problems. Officers are also influenced by life behind the perimeters, to the extent that many, of all ages, have consulted me in my private psychiatric practice, some of them with serious problems.

There is a stress condition among officers which I call "prison fatigue." It has four phases: anxiety, control, boredom and indifference. The average twenty-four-year-old recruit has no particular traumatic experiences. Usually he has chosen prison work for financial and job stability, having made other work starts with limited success. The problems begin occurring from the fifth to eighth year of service.

The phase of anxiety is one of reactive stresses and strikes when the officer is between twenty-eight and thirty-five years old and in the midst of supporting a young family. Conscious of his role as wage-earner, he frequently develops a state of anxiety and concern.

There are symptoms of sleeplessness, irritability and restlesseness. The anxieties are then reflected in his correctional duties and they are magnified in tense prison situations. Side symptoms involve marital quarrels, money problems, in-law difficulties and child discipline. Psychiatric attention in this phase is directed at stress handling, a type of coaching to assist, direct and encourage the officer to make use of simpler methods of coping with his stress. Frequently, a three to six month leave will provide him with time to adjust to his situation.

The second phase, "control," is a comfortable, accepting period in which the officer maintains his efficiency, at work and at home. But as the officer moves towards his fifteenth year of service, he begins to react to the dangers of his work. Threads of anxiety, nervousness, irritability and depression may appear. This reactive emotional state usually has no single stress factor (such as having been taken hostage). It is diagnosed by the officer as a feeling of discomfort. The condition is aggravated by new orders or plans, or changes in policy, which seem to disturb the stable function of the person.

In this phase, any change of routine is threatening and concerning.

Officers who have worked from twelve to fifteen years usually develop feelings of depression. They will say things like, "I'm going to pack it in," or "I can't handle the changes." At this point, I can identify the development of "morbid boredom", a condition which requires a period of three to six months sick leave. I attempt to eliminate their frustrations by getting them to accept their particular situations. With supportive counselling, they usually are able to return to their work and perform effectively.

Sometime after their fifteenth year of service (and before their twenty-fifth,) they enter the phase of "indifference," with signs of work fatigue and a diminished capability for physical exertion. While their experience is invaluable, these men, now between fifty and sixty years of age, find little excitement, or even interest, in their work. Emotionally and mentally, they develop a kind of passivity. They resent shift work, have difficulty handling commotion, resent new philosophies and techniques and generally feel too old for their jobs.

Certainly correctional officers are preoccupied with thoughts of retirement in the last few years of their service, but they still manage to function in a faithful way. I have a great deal of admiration for them.

A great many changes have occurred in our institutions during recent years and these have influenced the working lives of officers. They are, in fact, a different group of men today. The tight discipline of the early years (prior to 1960) produced strongly-motivated, prideful officers. The more permissive discipline of the last ten years has spread a feeling of insecurity and isolation in correctional ranks.

There has been a program of liberalization spawned by the civil rights movement, and in terms of social, political and legislative matters, inmates have become important people in the system. They have gained a great many concessions. They have a direct channel to members of

Parliament, a contact privilege denied the average man. A strong grievance can result in a headquarters investigation. Inmates can demand or refuse medical treatment and, in some cases, can almost dictate their treatment. They can be profane, rude and demanding and still have their allegations considered in Federal Government offices, by people, mind you, who have no real awareness, or understanding, of inmate mentality and motivation.

The young officers are growing up with the new thinking in prison administration. They accept the new expectations of management, the new heavy load of documentation that is required, the new thought and consideration given to inmates. My case records of men in their last years of service, however, present a different picture.

"With my grade eight education, it's hard keeping up with all the new directives," one man says.

"I can still handle an emergency," another says, "but it's having to spend a whole eight hours in there that bothers me."

"Sometimes it's so bad I think I'm going to cry," complains still another. "I try to keep it locked up inside. It's nuts. I was depressed six years ago when there was all that trouble in the joint with booze and pills. My depression is better now that I've had a leave but I have to be godamned careful that someday I don't just crack up the middle."

Many of the men who have come to me for counselling have complained about having to adjust to new administrative policies, but basically all of them realize that change is necessary, that it is a vital component of progress. The fact is, of course, that sooner or later, the joint gets to you. Sooner or later, you start getting jumpy. Sooner or later, you start looking over your shoulder when you walk among a bunch of inmates.

I won't soon forget the nervous officer who came to me for medication. He had to have something, he said, before he blew up. He was wringing his hands and his facial muscles were twitching as I wrote the prescription.

"Joe got it on the head," he said, the words coming slowly. "With an iron bar. It was this kooky inmate. There was no warning. I'm sorry for Joe, but do you know what I keep thinking Doc? I keep thinking...it could have been me."

**CHAPTER 23**

# Reward City: A New Penal Environment

Man, in his search for order and predictability, has developed standards of behavior which are basic to his survival and that of the society in which he lives. Infractions against the social order are defined as criminal acts and, as such, are punishable.

Each society develops its particular sanctions to meet its special needs. Time is the major governing factor since the changing patterns of life in each century drastically change the nature of criminal law and the punishment it prescribes.

The British system of justice, which governs our own, has undergone a number of major changes. It is interesting, going back to the first half of the eighteenth century, for example, to note that imprisonment was a temporary experience, a prelude to some other appropriate type of punishment. There were three categories of punishment at that time. One was debasement by means of whipping and placement in pillory (in some cases offenders were chained to the walls;) the second was death by public hanging, a sentence given for a myriad of offences from theft to murder; and the third, for frequent and serious offenders, was deportation to far-off countries, notably the colonies in North America.

English records show that fourteen per cent of all punishments called for death; thirty-four per cent involved imprisonment with specific punishments; and fifty-two per cent prescribed deportation.

Security in the old English prisons was maintained by the simple process of chaining. The jail-keeper had complete authority over his charges with no supervision apart from a few turnkeys who attended the doors, admitted visitors and placed and removed irons as required. Internal order was enforced by the inmates' subcultural standards.

Not all prisons, of course, were places where offenders were held for specific punishments. There were debtors' prisons, for instance, where debtors and their families were confined until they could satisfy their creditors. There were county jails where felons facing trial, sentence, or execution were held pending disposition of their cases. There were also corrective institutions where efforts were made to put offenders to work at some skill or trade. Outside industries thus could contract with the jails to provide cheap labor.

Historical events have had their influence on prison concepts. The most notable, in terms of English justice, was the American Revolution of 1776 which effectively cut off deportation of felons to its shores. It was a paralyzing blow to a system which made use of deportation in more than half of all its criminal cases.

Australia provided a far-away home for deported individuals but could not replace the American colonies. The result was that new jails and penitentiaries had to be built to cope with all of the offenders who could no longer be deported. Massive structures were built between 1790 and 1850 with numerous designs based on cellular confinement.

Upper and Lower Canada followed the Americans, struggling with the massive new prison complex. The Canadian institutions were hewn from the English mother system, with massive, impregnable stone structures like Kingston Penitentiary and St. Vincent de Paul Penitentiary in Québec. With their massive fortress gates, small cells and stockade-like workshops, they soon became symbols of the new penology.

By 1840, imprisonment was no longer a temporary experience, or prelude to punishment. Imprisonment was punishment in itself, though floggings, even of women and children, continued. Life behind bars was made as uncomfortable and irksome as possible. Starvation diets were introduced. Treadmills were installed as a thoroughly monotonous form of useless hard labor. The rule of sentence had become uniform, with solitary confinement the final step in discomfort and discipline.

The militarization of guards became necessary to limit the abuses of previous jailers. Guards were drilled, uniformed and indoctrinated with the serious responsibilities of their calling. They were also placed on regular pay and forbidden to associate (as their predecessors had done) with street felons.

The new prisons were awesome places. They also were places of great curiosity. Officials of Kingston Penitentiary, aware of a public morbidity for such matters, allowed the public to visit the building at any time. Male adults were charged 1 shilling, 3 pence and women and children 7 1/2 pence. It was a low-priced admission considering that the custodial circus was a continuous show.

What went on behind the walls in the early days would certainly shock people today. Yet, in the mid 1800's, no one thought it unusual to treat convicts harshly. One staff member even used a prisoner as a target in his bow-and-arrow practices.

While prison authorities held to the old concepts of punishment, however, other voices were urging a change in approach. One such voice was that of John Howard who sought reform in several areas of prison life, including the practice of solitary cellular confinement, constant supervision and the enforced hours of penitence-praying.

John Howard had introduced the philosophy of treatment of the criminal in the late 1700's, at a time when the big new prison complexes were springing up on both sides of the Atlantic. In the early 1800's, a woman named Elizabeth Fry aroused the interests of the Evangelical and Quaker movements with her belief that the reformation of criminals represented the triumph of God's grace. Between 1816 and 1832, she carried out a highly successful program of reform among women prisoners in the jails of England.

John and Elizabeth, of course, could have had no idea of the legacy they were leaving for future generations. They sowed the seeds of reform and laid the groundwork for a penal philosophy that surprised even the reformers. I think they would be shocked if they walked into one of our present-day institutions and saw what has replaced the treadmills and the starvation diets.

**As it is now**

Each penitentiary system is dependant upon prosecution under the Criminal Code and the court system for its flow of inmates. While the law is designed to be fair and just, it can be interpreted as less fair and more unjust in certain circumstances.

The prevalence of a specific type of criminal act, the intensity with which the police apply the rules of law, the speed and effectiveness of the criminal courts – all affect the conviction process. Wise and human men on the Bench may also err at times, not in matters of law but in their own very personal attitudes toward different kinds of offences and offenders.

Yet, it is surprising how many inmates arrive in prison with nothing more than the odd remark in passing about their trials. There is no enmity for the judge of prosecutor. And there is no interest in the jury collectively, or in the juror individually.

To most new inmates, the whole court procedure is a game of chance. It's like playing a slot machine. You pull the crank, wait expectantly and accept the consequences of the gamble.

Inmates have no standards by which they can judge the efficiency and effectiveness of their counsel. I am reminded of two cases with which I was concerned recently. Both revolved around the death of a homosexual person, and in each case the offence data was similar. Because of a poor defence, one of the accused ended up with a life sentence. The second accused was represented by expert counsel and had his murder charge reduced to manslaughter, for which he was sentenced to eight years.

The Victorian concept has faded. Criminal man need no longer accept his guilt personally, or show penitent remorse for the offence. Now, the inmate's degree of irritation over his imprisonment overwhelms the balance of judgment. He no longer talks in terms of "What have I done?" Rather, he asks, "What are they trying to do to me?"

Inmates, however, have a passive, unspoken acceptance of the justification of imprisonment. If this were not so, the prison society could, at any time, take over each and every institution by force and hold it for a considerable period of time. As it is, prisoners may (and do,) under aggravating and provoking conditions, resist commands, conduct strikes, take hostages and stage destructive, attention-getting riots. Interestingly enough, every prison riot has centered around some internal, domestic problem which was unresolved. Problems include over-crowding, inadequate food, unreasonable discipline, administrative inconsistencies and unexpected changes in an inmate's life.

The old theories and concepts of the nineteenth century have pretty well all been discarded and today inmates are able to seek redress for any legitimate problem. They can take their grievances to court, claiming cruel and unjust treatment, contrary to the Canadian Bill of Rights.

I sat for two weeks in a court in British Columbia where a class action of ten inmates was heard by a justice of the Supreme Court of Canada. The judge upheld the action of the inmates, concluding that indeed there had been cruel and unjust treatment. The action resulted in a systematic review of all segregation and solitary confinement regulations.

The Canadian prison system has responded quietly to the ground swells of progressive and humanizing improvements. Canada has never been known as an innovator of concepts but it has been wise enough to adopt practices developed in other countries, among them the half way house (to bridge the traumatic period between imprisonment and freedom,) the conjugal visiting system and similar steps to reduce the solitary ill-effects of prison.

**As it will be**

The shape of time dictates the adjustment of society. The American Revolution destroyed the deportation process, forcing England to develop large-scale prisons as punitive centres in the early 1800's. Now, the exceptionally high cost of labor and supplies is forcing the Canadian prison system to adopt new principles of incarceration with a view to reducing operational costs while maintaining a high degree of custodial effectiveness.

It is estimated that it costs $80 per day to feed, house, train and supervise each inmate. This represents a yearly cost factor of $29,000 per inmate, and with some 9,000 offenders behind bars, it means an annual bill of well over $261,000,000.

It is likely that mounting costs will bring about drastic changes in our philosophy, just as the American Revolution produced unexpected changes in the English system. The following are suggestions for remedying the cost problem:

1. New sentence alternatives

At present, individuals sentenced to two years or more are sent to federal penitentiaries, while those with sentences of less than two years serve their time in provincial jails. I suggest that the minimum sentence for admission to the federal system be increased to four years. (The regulations now state that, with good behavior, an inmate serves seven-tenths of his sentence, with parole eligibility considered yearly.) For sentences of less than four years, social alternatives to imprisonment have to be found in areas of federal and provincial government projects, wherein probates would receive minimum wages in return for their labors.

2. Social compliance and danger factor

All inmates should be assessed in terms of their danger potential. Fifty per cent of offenders under twenty-five years of age have varying degrees of impulsivity, are potentially dangerous and are security risks in nearly all situations. Older inmates, those between twenty-five and forty, have greater emotional control and can accept minimal security care as long as labor and industrial workshops give them financial incentives. Many offenders show no danger signs, though their crimes reflect extremely aggressive behavior, due usually to a particular set of circumstances. Eighty per cent of murderers show no ongoing problems of an emotional or mental nature. Seventy-five per cent of manslaughters have developed from situations which initially were not criminal. In these cases, minimal security institutions provide sufficient supervision and promote a feeling of inherent trust among inmates.

3. Subsidized parole

Individuals with a prison record have a discouraging role in society, not unlike that of unemployed citizens who fret about their abilities as workers. These ex-inmates need financial help until the prison confusion leaves them and street orientation establishes itself. Not all parolees need help but a high percentage do, and considering the $80-a-day cost of keeping a man in prison, a release payment of $20 a day is a financial bargain for the authorities. My concept is that parolees should have help for the first three to six months after release.

I have known many inmates with wives and children who have gotten into trouble after leaving prison because of finances. Mothers' allowances had helped the families while the men were in prison, but stopped as soon as they were freed. The result was that the families were plunged into want and debt and the men went back to crime.

4. Disability pensions

These have played an important role in helping physically, mentally and emotionally disabled people to carry on in society with a degree of independence and self-respect. I believe that ten per cent of inmates are totally disabled because of their mental and emotional problems and leave prison only to return anxiously because adequate care is available to them all the time. They have no trade, only limited education and no motivation. A social disability is as specific and obvious as a physical or mental one. Long-time, state-supported persons with records of incarceration since youth, have limited social skills and few financial resources. These people must be made eligible for provincial disability pensions.

5. Advocate parole courts

Long-term inmates should have full opportunity to plead their cases in a court of law. It is generally accepted now that individuals who have spent ten solid years in prison require encouragement and social activation, with some firm hope of eventual release. In the envisioned parole court they are given a chance to show that they are ready to return to society. In court, inmates are represented by prisoner advocates who may call witnesses from among penitentiary staff, public bodies and families of the individuals concerned. Parole advocates, on the other hand, act as prosecution lawyers, examining and cross-examining to clarify questions of motivation and the ability of prisoners to adapt to life outside. Cases are heard by five-member juries, made up from county jury lists.

These suggestions deal prisoners a material advantage. They also reduce the prohibitive – and constantly rising – cost of caring for them.

Sentence restructuring reduces the number of admissions to the main prison system by introducing farm, industrial and work camp environments. A minimum security camp is built at smaller capital cost and requires reduced maintenance and security. This represents a calculated per diem drop from $80 per day to $50.

Subsidized parole is a maintenance allowance for a specified period of time to assist inmates to adapt socially to free society and to help them in trade or academic training. Parole revocations and re-entry into prisons would be reduced as crime flows naturally from unemployment and poverty.

Disability pensions for the mentally and emotionally disturbed would reduce their criminality markedly. Crimes among these people usually are poorly planned with a minimum amount of aggressiveness.

Sometimes as I drive along the highway, I imagine I can see a sign. reading "Reward City." It's pure imagination, of course. There is no sign. There is no "Reward City." But someday, I tell myself, it will exist. Someday there will be such a place.

Right now, "Reward City" is a concept, an idea for a progressive, productive prison program that has lain dormant in my notes for nearly fifteen years. I thought it was a practical workable plan when I wrote about it in "The Psychodynamics of the Captive" back in the 1960's. I still think so.

"Reward City" is my name for a total prison community – a city for inmates and their families, a place where prisoners would prepare themselves for re-entry into free society.

I am not the only one to have thought along these lines. Thomas Murton, of the Department of Criminal Justice, University of Minnesota, envisioned a similar complex. Swedish progressives acquired an abandoned lumbering village in 1972 and used it as an experimental home for prisoners and their families. In Illinois, the Vienna Correctional Centre, a minimum security institution, was designed on the village concept, with nineteen buildings around a town square.

"Reward City" would be a total prison complex, involving medium and minimum security systems and including a combined service hospital with medical, surgical and psychiatric facilities. There would be a three-storey peripheral building for administrative and civic functions; six three-storey apartment buildings for inmate occupancy; a food services building strategically placed near the living area; a gymnasium and civic theatre with library; and several large service buildings housing the fire department and building trade shops. There would also be an indoor rink, swimming pool and bowling alley, so important for the physical retraining of inmates. Included in the civic centre would be a chapel. Nearby would be a courtroom with adjoining legal offices.

The whole complex would be organized on an oval-based paved road with an urban transit system of transportation around the area. There would be no motor vehicles. Computer-operated transit cars would be the fixed transportation facility.

I visualize my city not only as a living area but also in terms of providing employment for inmates. I can see federally supported corporations setting up shops in a great circle surrounding the oval. I can see inmates reporting for a wide variety of jobs each day and getting reasonable wages for their efforts.

An impossible dream? Not at all. I have worked out the plans in detail. It's a workable scheme. I have even chosen a possible site. I am convinced that the Millhaven Institution area could be made to function as "Reward City" with the simple addition of shops, civic buildings and labor facilities of Crown corporations.

The Canadian prison system has been described as progressive and yet conservative. That may be a fair assessment. Those of us who work in the institutions – and perhaps even those who are confined in them – have a quota of petty grievances, but I think we'd all have to admit that the level of care is adequately high. I believe we live up to standards as high as any progressive country in the world.

That is not to say that we haven't a long way to go still. But you have to look out of the back window to see how far you've come.

I become acutely aware of the progress we have made every time I walk through the gates of Kingston Penitentiary. There are very few prisoners there now – just psychiatric cases and inmates awaiting transfer to another institution. Some day, I hope, there will only be ghosts.

# APPENDIX I
# POPULATION PROFILE REPORT

A statistical study of the inmate population in federal and provincial institutions in Canada

| 1. Population by age | <16 | 16 | 17 | 18 | 19 | 20-24 | 25-29 | 30-34 | 35-39 | 40-44 | 45-49 | 50-59 | 60-64 | 65 + |
|---|---|---|---|---|---|---|---|---|---|---|---|---|---|---|
| Number | 0 | 1 | 35 | 119 | 269 | 2,657 | 2,357 | 1,719 | 953 | 587 | 383 | 354 | 56 | 55 |
| Percentage | 0.00 | 0.01 | 0.36 | 1.24 | 2.81 | 27.83 | 24.69 | 18.00 | 9.98 | 6.14 | 4.01 | 3.70 | 0.58 | 0.57 |

| 2. Major Offence Analysis | Murder | Attempted Murder | Manslaughter | Rape | Other Sexual Offences | Kidnapping & Abduction | Wounding | Assault |
|---|---|---|---|---|---|---|---|---|
| Number | 1,091 | 206 | 550 | 516 | 210 | 147 | 165 | 108 |
| Percentage | 11.43 | 2.15 | 5.76 | 5.40 | 2.20 | 1.54 | 1.72 | 1.13 |
| | Robbery | Offensive Weapons | Prison Breach | Break & Enter | Theft | Possession of Stolen Goods | Fraud | Criminal Negligence |
| Number | 2,584 | 126 | 33 | 1,323 | 287 | 189 | 267 | 34 |
| Percentage | 27.07 | 1.32 | 0.34 | 13.86 | 3.00 | 1.98 | 2.79 | 0.35 |
| | Dangerous Sex Offenders | Habitual Criminal | Dangerous Offenders | Other Offences Criminal Code | Narcotics | Food & Drug Act | Other Statutes | |
| Number | 52 | 32 | 0 | 794 | 801 | 0 | 30 | |
| Percentage | 0.54 | 0.33 | 0.00 | 8.31 | 8.39 | 0.00 | 0.31 | |

| 3. Length of Sentence | <2 | 2-3 | 3-4 | 4-5 | 5-6 | 6-10 | 10-15 | 15-20 | 20 + | Preventive Detention | Life | Indefinite |
|---|---|---|---|---|---|---|---|---|---|---|---|---|
| Number | 594 | 1,793 | 1,474 | 967 | 756 | 1,422 | 736 | 285 | 180 | 121 | 1,210 | 7 |
| Percentage | 6.22 | 18.78 | 15.44 | 10.13 | 7.92 | 14.89 | 7.71 | 2.98 | 1.88 | 1.26 | 12.67 | 0.0 |

| 4. No. of Previous Commitments | 0 | 1 | 2 | 3 | 4 | 5 | 6 | 7 | 8 | 9 | 10-15 | 16-20 | 20 + |
|---|---|---|---|---|---|---|---|---|---|---|---|---|---|
| Number | 5,791 | 2,056 | 933 | 431 | 207 | 76 | 27 | 17 | 5 | 1 | 1 | 0 | 0 |
| **Percentage** | 60.67 | 21.54 | 9.77 | 4.51 | 2.16 | 0.79 | 0.28 | 0.17 | 0.05 | 0.01 | 0.01 | 0.00 | 0.00 |

| 5. Marital Status | Single | Married | Common Law | Widowed | Separated | Divorced | Not Stated |
|---|---|---|---|---|---|---|---|
| Number | 5,171 | 1,426 | 1,879 | 135 | 401 | 499 | 34 |
| Percentage | 54.17 | 14.93 | 19.68 | 1.41 | 4.20 | 5.22 | 0.35 |

| 6. Race | Not Stated | Caucasian | North American Indian | Metis | Eskimo (Inuit) | Asiatic (Mongoloid) | Black (Negroid) | Other |
|---|---|---|---|---|---|---|---|---|
| Number | 322 | 8,092 | 594 | 233 | 24 | 61 | 186 | 43 |
| Percentage | 3.37 | 84.77 | 6.22 | 2.33 | 0.25 | 0.63 | 1.94 | 0.4 |

| 7. Language Spoken | English | French | Both | Neither | 8. Citizenship | Canadian | U.S. | Other |
|---|---|---|---|---|---|---|---|---|
| | [illegible] | [illegible] | [illegible] | 47 | | 9,137 | 120 | 288 |
| | | | | | | [illegible] | [illegible] | [illegible] |

| | | | | | | | |
|---|---|---|---|---|---|---|---|
| | [illegible] | [illegible] | 31.01 | 0.03 | 1.19 | 57.20 | 3.14 |

| 10. Province of Residence | Not Stated | NFLD | P.E.I. | Nova Scotia | New Brunswick | Quebec | Ontario |
|---|---|---|---|---|---|---|---|
| Number | 388 | 174 | 28 | 406 | 296 | 2,893 | 2,236 |
| Percentage | 4.06 | 1.82 | 0.29 | 4.25 | 3.10 | 30.30 | 23.42 |
| | Manitoba | Sask | Alberta | B.C. | Yukon | N.W.T. | Outside of Canada |
| Number | 468 | 249 | 1,018 | 1,214 | 16 | 30 | 129 |
| Percentage | 4.90 | 2.60 | 10.66 | 12.71 | 0.16 | 0.31 | 1.35 |

| 11. Type of Admission | WARRANT OF COMMITTAL | PROVINCIAL TRANSFER SECTION 659 (5) | PAROLE REVOKED | PAROLE FORFEITED | PAROLE REVOKED WITH OFFENCE | MANDATORY SUPERVISION REVOKED | MANDATORY SUPERVISION FOREITED | MANDATORY SUPERVISION REVOKED WITH OFFENCE | FED PROV CONTRACT | OTHER |
|---|---|---|---|---|---|---|---|---|---|---|
| Number | 7,357 | 271 | 221 | 220 | 301 | 220 | 152 | 625 | 112 | 76 |
| Percentage | 77.07 | 2.83 | 2.21 | 2.30 | 3.15 | 2.30 | 1.59 | 6.54 | 1.17 | 0.79 |

| 12. Time Served | 0-3 MTH | 3 - 6 MTH | 6 - 9 MTH | 9 - 12 MTH | 12 - 18 MTH | 18 - 24 MTH | 2 - 3 YRS | 3 - 4 YRS | 4 - 5 YRS | 5 - 10 YRS | 10 plus YRS |
|---|---|---|---|---|---|---|---|---|---|---|---|
| Number | 938 | 639 | 956 | 894 | 1,223 | 1,161 | 1,287 | 701 | 428 | 976 | 343 |
| Percentage | 9.82 | 6.68 | 10.01 | 9.36 | 12.81 | 12.16 | 13.48 | 7.34 | 4.48 | 10.22 | 3.5 |

| 13. Time in Inst. since last transfer | 0 - 1 MTH | 1 - 2 MTH | 2 - 3 MTH | 3 - 6 MTH | 6 - 9 MTH | 9 - 12 MTH | 12 - 18 MTH | 18 - 24 MTH | 2 - 3 YRS | 3 - 4 YRS | 4 - 5 YRS | 5 plus YRS |
|---|---|---|---|---|---|---|---|---|---|---|---|---|
| Number | 0 | 356 | 311 | 1,073 | 1,500 | 1,936 | 2,220 | 966 | 623 | 235 | 117 | 208 |
| Percentage | 0.00 | 3.72 | 3.25 | 11.24 | 15.71 | 20.28 | 23.25 | 10.12 | 6.52 | 2.46 | 1.22 | 2.1 |

14. Probable Mandatory Supervision release date by quarter within calendar year

| Quarter | 1980 | 1980 | 1981 | 1982 | 1983 | 1984 | 1985 | 1986 | 1987 | 1988 | 1989 | 1990 | 1991 | 1992 | 1993 | 1994 | 1995 | 1995 | 1997 | 1997 | INDF | LIFE | PD |
|---|---|---|---|---|---|---|---|---|---|---|---|---|---|---|---|---|---|---|---|---|---|---|---|
| 1 | 42 | 749 | 752 | 294 | 173 | 117 | 66 | 48 | 32 | 16 | 14 | 6 | 9 | 2 | 0 | 3 | 1 | 1 | 1 | 5 | 38 | 1,209 | 121 |
| 2 | 47 | 704 | 649 | 301 | 147 | 105 | 59 | 31 | 21 | 11 | 13 | 6 | 4 | 3 | 2 | 4 | 1 | 2 | 1 | 1 | 0 | 0 | 0 |
| 3 | 57 | 745 | 439 | 231 | 127 | 92 | 56 | 24 | 14 | 17 | 8 | 8 | 3 | 1 | 2 | 1 | 1 | 0 | 0 | 3 | 0 | 0 | 0 |
| 4 | 112 | 731 | 453 | 205 | 129 | 68 | 56 | 28 | 25 | 13 | 10 | 8 | 6 | 2 | 4 | 0 | 1 | 1 | 0 | 3 | 0 | 0 | 0 |
| TOTAL | 258 | 2929 | 2343 | 1031 | 576 | 382 | 237 | 131 | 92 | 57 | 45 | 28 | 22 | 8 | 8 | 8 | 4 | 4 | 2 | 12 | 38 | 1,209 | 121 |

*** Total number of inmates processed in Federal and Provincial Institutions: 9,545

(PRODUCED BY INFORMATION SERVICES, CORRECTIONAL SERVICES CANADA JANUARY 1981)

# APPENDIX II

## Inmates' Rights Handbook

# FOREWORD

The Correctional Service of Canada accepts the basic proposition that an inmate retains all of the rights of an ordinary citizen save those which have been removed either by law, or by the necessary implication of incarceration. The Correctional Service of Canada also accepts, as a basic principle, the fact that the sentence which the Court has imposed on an inmate should constitute his only punishment. The Correctional Service of Canada will not impose additional penalties except for disciplinary offences for which an inmate has been found guilty by a properly established administrative tribunal. Discipline and order will be maintained with firmness, but with no more restriction than is necessary for safe custody and well-ordered community life.

This Handbook is a collection of the more important rights of which you, as an inmate, may avail yourself. They are of three basic kinds, what we have called "Retained Rights", "Existing Rights in the Penitentiary Act and Regulations" and "Conferred Rights":

(a) Retained Rights are those deriving either from our system and tradition of common law or laws of Parliament which you share with all citizens of Canada, to the extent that they have not been specifically taken away, either by law, or by the necessary implications of your imprisonment. Obviously, any such list cannot be exhaustive and you will find reference only to those rights which may be of significant importance to you as an inmate.

(b) Existing Rights in the Penitentiary Act and Regulations are those specific rights which have been granted to you as an inmate, by Parliament or by the Government and for which you may seek redress from the Courts if you feel they have been denied you. In most cases, these are rights which are unique to inmates and are not shared with other members of Canadian society.

(c) Conferred Rights are those which have been specifically granted to you as an inmate, by the Commissioner, by virtue of the power given to him by Parliament in section 29 (3) of the Penitentiary Act, to make rules, known as Commissioner's Directives. If you feel that you have been denied one of these "Conferred Rights" or that it has been unfairly applied to you, you may seek redress through the grievance system of The Correctional Service of Canada, which is described in Commissioner's Directive No. 241 and in the Inmate Grievance Manual, both of which are available in your library. You should also be aware of the Directive relating to privileged correspondence and of the existence of the Correctional Investigator of Canada.

In some cases, Retained and Existing rights are applied without restriction. In most cases, however, these rights are unavoidably limited by other laws or regulations, which exist to safeguard the rights of many other people.

In this light, you should also realize that provision of certain services to you must be based on reasonable standards and expectations. If you have been convicted of a disciplinary offence, for example, you cannot expect to take advantage of all the rights available to your fellow inmates. In cases of disturbances or disruptions of normal institutional life, the responsibility of The Correctional Service of Canada to protect you, other inmates and the public, may override the application of certain rights. Ultimately, you alone can ensure that you remain in a position to take advantage of all of the benefits to which you feel you are entitled. If you behave unreasonably, you can only expect restrictions, limitations or perhaps even curtailment of the rights which are set out in this manual.

Finally, you should remember that this document, while an official Correctional Service of Canada publication, is only a consolidation drawn from many sources - sources of either an administrative or legal nature which have been brought together in order to make you aware of your rights. It is not in itself a legal document and has no force as such. It you wish to make a grievance concerning the application of a "Conferred Right", you should base your complaint on the actual Commissioner's Directive itself and not on the Handbook.

July 1980

# DISCRIMINATION

1. Every inmate has the right:

   (a) to be free from any discrimination related to the prohibitions contained in the Canadian Human Rights Act.

   (Retained)

   Reference: Canadian Human Rights Act 3,5 to 13

   (b) to file a complaint with the Human Rights Commission when he has reasonable grounds to believe that a person is engaging or has engaged in a discriminatory practice.

   (Retained)

   Reference: Canadian Human Rights Act 4,32

# LANGUAGE

2. Every inmate has the right, in accordance with the rules set out in Commissioner's Directives:

   (a) to retain all language rights assured to the community at large by the Official Languages Act.

   (Retained)

   Reference: Official Languages Act
   CD 237

(b) to choose either English or French as his preferred official language and to use the official language he has chosen in his dealings with The Correctional Service of Canada unless the security of the general public, the inmate population or the personnel of the Service is jeopardized.

(Retained)

Reference: Official Languages Act
CD 237

(c) to appeal to the Commissioner of Official Languages if he feels his language rights are not being respected.

(Retained)

Reference: Official Languages Act
PSR 13

(d) to use his own language, whether or not it is one of the two official languages, in his correspondence, with his visitors, and with other inmates unless security considerations make this impossible.

(Conferred)

Reference: CD 226

(e) When he is unable to speak and understand either of the two official languages, to be provided the assistance of an interpreter, especially in disciplinary hearings.

(Conferred)

Reference: CD 226

# FEMALE INMATES

3. (a) Female inmates have the same rights as male inmates and an equal opportunity to earn privileges, within the limits of the institutions' resources.

(Retained)

Reference: Canadian Human Rights Act

(b) No female inmate shall be kept in a form of custody in which, without the constant supervision of an officer, she can associate with male persons.

(Existing)

Reference: PSR 24

(c) Where the institutional head suspects, on reasonable grounds, that an officer, employee, inmate or visitor to the institution is in possession of contraband, he may order that person to be searched, but no such person, who is female, shall be searched except by a female person.

(Existing)

Reference: PSR 41 (2)

(d) Female inmates shall have obstetric delivery done at an outside hospital, wherever practicable.

(Conferred)

Reference: CD 226

# CONFIDENTIALITY

4. Every inmate and former inmate,

(a) has access to records containing personal information concerning him for the purposes listed in Section 52 (1) of the Canadian Human Rights Act.

(Retained)

Reference: Canadian Human Rights Act 52 (1)

(b) will be advised in writing by the appropriate Minister, when his rights under Section 51 (1) of the Act are denied on the ground that, by virtue of Section 54 or 55, Section 52 (1) or a provision thereof does not apply in the circumstances, of the particular ground on which the right is denied.

(Retained)

Reference: Canadian Human Rights Act 52 (4)

(c) will have CSC records concerning him/her kept confidential, and the information therein shall not be disclosed to any person except as authorized by directives.

(Existing)

Reference: PSR 23

(d) is entitled to be consulted and must consent before personal information concerning him that was provided by him to a government institution for a particular purpose is used or made available for use for any non-derivative use for an administrative purpose unless the use of that information for that non-derivative use is authorized by or pursuant to law. Where notice in writing is given to an individual that personal information described above concerning that individual is proposed to be used for a purpose specified in the notice that is a non-derivative use for an administrative purpose, that individual shall be deemed to have been consulted and to have consented to the use of the information for the specified purpose unless written notice to the contrary is given by the individual, in a prescribed manner and within a prescribed time specified in the notice.

(Retained)

Reference: Canadian Human Rights Act 52 (2) and (3)

(e) is entitled to complain to the Privacy Commissioner of the Human Rights Commission when he believes that he is not being accorded the rights to which he is entitled under Part IV of the Act in relation to personal information concerning him that is recorded in a federal information bank.

(Retained)

Reference: Canadian Human Rights Act 58

# RECEPTION

5. (a) A person who has been sentenced or committed to a penitentiary shall not be received in a penitentiary until after the expiration of the time limited by law for an appeal and thereupon be received in a penitentiary whether or not he has entered an appeal; but any such person may, before the expiration of the time limited by law for an appeal, give written notice, in the Court that sentenced or committed him, that he elects not to appeal or abandons his appeal, as the case may be, and thereupon the time limited for appeal shall be deemed to have expired.

(Existing)

Reference: Penitentiary Act 16 (1)

(b) The institutional head shall take reasonable care to ensure that the effects of an inmate, which in accordance with directives, he is permitted to bring into and keep in the institution, are protected from loss or damage.

(Existing)

Reference: PSR 18

# CLASSIFICATION

6. (a) Every inmate shall, in accordance with directives, be confined in the institution that seems most appropriate having regard to:

(i) the degree and kind of custodial control considered necessary or desirable for the protection of society, and
(ii) the program of correctional training considered most appropriate for the inmate.

(Existing)

Reference: PSR 13

(b) The file of an inmate shall be carefully reviewed before any decision is made concerning the classification, reclassification or transfer of the inmate.

(Existing)

Reference: PSR 14

# ACCOMMODATION AND ESSENTIAL SERVICES

7. (a) It is the duty of the institutional head to take all reasonable steps to ensure the safe custody of inmates committed to his care.

(Existing)

Reference: PSR 37

(b) Consideration shall be given to providing inmates with standards of accommodation which meet the requirements of health.

(Conferred)

Reference: CD 226

(c) Every inmate shall be:
   (i) adequately fed and clothed, according to the requirements of the season and the nature of his employment, and
   (ii) provided with adequate bedding.

(Existing)

Reference: PSR 15 (1)

(d) No inmate shall be required to wear clothing that, by its nature, is calculated to subject him to ridicule or contempt from other persons.

(Existing)

Reference: PSR 15 (2)

(e) Toilet articles and other articles necessary for personal health and cleanliness shall be issued to every inmate.

(Existing)

Reference: PSR 17

(f) (i) Every inmate is entitled, where weather permits, to a daily period of exercise in the open air, in accordance with directives.

(Existing)

Reference: PSR 19

(ii) The period of exercise mentioned above shall be of one hour's duration, weather, operational conditions and security considerations permitting.

(Conferred)

Reference: CD 226

(iii) An effort shall be made to have physicial or recreational training equipment available during those periods.

(Conferred)

Reference: CD 226

# HEALTH CARE

8. (a) Every inmate shall be provided, in accordance with directives, with the essential medical and dental care that he requires.

(Existing)

Reference: PSR 16

(b) Every inmate shall have his request for health care conveyed to the health staff without undue delay and without exception.

(Conferred)

Reference: CD 226

(c) Every inmate may request elective surgery or treatment and shall have such requests given due consideration.

(Conferred)

Reference: CD 226

(d) Inmates shall not be subjected, without their full, free and informed consent, to any form of medical or scientific experimentation, and may at any time, discontinue their participation in any medical research project.

(Retained)

Reference: Common Law

(e) Every inmate, if he is deemed to be competent, may refuse any prescribed medical care, including hospitalization, preventive measures, tests or examinations, except when these are mandatory under law, or the condition is a threat to life.

(Retained)

Reference: Common Law

(f) Every inmate shall be informed of the reasons for, and consent to, medical examinations for purposes of classification, parole, or prison discipline, or for similar purposes. A body cavity search ordered by the institutional head or senior duty officer for security purposes does not constitute a medical examination.

(Retained)

Reference: Common Law

N.B. Health care rights a, b, and c pertain only to inmates who are incarcerated or on day parole, not to inmates on other forms of parole or under mandatory supervision.

# INFORMATION FOR INMATES

9. Every inmate has the right,

(a) to be provided with all necessary written information concerning the conditions under which he is to serve his sentence, and if he is illiterate, to have this information conveyed to him orally. He is to be given a copy of his sentence computation sheet and he is to be shown his warrant of committal.

(Conferred)

Reference: CD 226

(b) to have access to a library, at every institution adequately stocked, and containing copies of

(i) specified Statutes and Regulations to which he may need to refer,
(ii) the Commissioner's Directives dealing with the treatment and training of inmates, and
(iii) the Index of Federal Information Banks.

(Conferred)

Reference: CD 226

# RELIGION

10. Every inmate has the right,
(a) to freedom of religion.

(Retained)

Reference: Canadian Bill of Rights

(b) to be free from coercion which would impair his freedom to have or to adopt a religion or belief of his choice.

(Retained)

Reference: Canadian Bill of Rights

(c) to manifest his religion or belief in worship and observance of practice, individually or in community with others, subject only to the requirements of safety and security, and of the good order and administration of the institution.

(Conferred)

Reference: CD 226

(d) to have in his possession, subject to the requirements of PSR 31, the books of religious observance and instruction of his denomination or faith.

(Conferred)

Reference: CD 209, Annex A

(e) where practical, to be allowed visits by a qualified representative of his stated religion, unless denial is clearly required in the interests of safety or security, or of the good order and administration of the institution. Such visits shall be approved by the institutional head or his delegate and coordinated by the institutional Chaplain.

(Conferred)

Reference: CD 226

(f) No inmate shall be compelled, against his wishes, to participate in religious activities.

(Existing)

Reference: PSR 20(3)

# PROGRAMS GENERALLY

11. (a) (i) There shall be, at each institution, an appropriate program of in-

mate activities designed, as far as practicable, to prepare inmates, upon discharge, to assume their responsibilities as citizens and to conform to the requirements of the law.

(ii) For the purpose of giving effect to subsection (1), the Commissioner shall, so far as practicable, make available to each inmate who is capable of benefitting therefrom, academic or vocational training, instructive and productive work, religious and recreational activities and psychiatric, psychological and social counselling.

(Existing)

Reference: PSR 20 (1) and (2)

(b) No inmate shall be compelled against his wishes to parcicipate in recreational or religious activities.

(Existing)

Reference: PSR 20 (3)

(c) Inmates may buy or subscribe to newspapers, magazines and books.

(Conferred)

Reference: CD 215

(d) No reading material, of any description, shall be permitted in an institution if it is calculated:

(i ) to bring into ridicule or contempt any religion or faith,

(ii ) to promote controversy between members of different religions or faiths,

(iii) to affect adversely the good order or administration of the institution.

(Existing)

Reference: PSR 31

(e) Every inmate shall have access to a library, at every institution, adequately stocked with materials of an educational, cultural and recreational nature.

(Conferred)

Reference: CD 226

(f) The visiting and correspondence privileges that may, in accordance with directives, be permitted to inmates shall be such as are, in all the circumstances, calculated to assist in the reformation and rehabilitation of the inmate.

(Existing)

Reference: PSR 27

(g) In so far as practicable, the censorship of correspondence shall be avoided and the privacy of visits shall be maintained, but nothing herein shall be deemed to limit the authority of the Commissioner to direct or the institutional head to order censorship of correspondence or supervision of visiting to the extent considered necessary or desirable for the reformation and rehabilitation of inmates or the security of the institution.

(Existing)

Reference: PSR 28

# EDUCATIONAL, VOCATIONAL TRAINING AND WORK

12. Every inmate is required to work at an occupation or activity that is calculated to assist in his reformation and rehabilitation.

(a) Sundays and statutory holidays are not working days except for inmates who, on those days, are required to perform necessary administrative tasks or to meet an emergency.

(Existing)

Reference: PSR 35 (2)

(b) To conform with work conditions in the community at large, Saturdays are not working days except for inmates, who, on those days, are required to perform necessary administrative tasks or to meet an emergency.

(Conferred)

Reference: CD 226

(c) No inmate shall be required to work for the personal benefit of any private person.

(Existing)

Reference: PSR 35 (3)

(d) No inmate shall be employed in a disciplinary capacity over another inmate.

(Existing)

Reference: PSR 35 (4)

(e) Where an inmate alleges that he is not physically fit to perform the work to which he has been assigned, he shall not be employed at that work unless the physician certifies that he is physically fit to perform it.

(Existing)

Reference: PSR 35 (5)

(f) Insofar as possible, an inmate's wishes shall be given full consideration in deciding the type of occupation or activity to which he will be assigned.

(Conferred)

References: CD 221
CD 236

(g) Every inmate shall be kept actively employed in the work, training or educational activities that he is required to carry out, for the full institutional working day, wherever practicable.

(Conferred)

References: CD 221
CD 236

(h) While educational opportunities are available to all inmates, special attention shall be given to providing basic education to inmates who are illiterate or under the age of 19, and are capable of benefitting from it.

(Conferred)

Reference: CD 226

# REMUNERATION AND INMATE TRUST FUND

13. (a) Every inmate shall receive remuneration for satisfactory performance in the authorized activities of the institutional program.

(Conferred)

Reference: CD 232

(b) Every inmate shall receive, while he is incarcerated, a basic allowance when he is unable, through no fault of his own, to work or engage in training, or when, except for disciplinary reasons, no work, training or education is available to him.

(Conferred)

Reference: CD 232

(c) All moneys that accompany an inmate to an institution and all moneys received on his behalf while he is in custody shall be deposited to his credit in a trust account to be known as the Inmate Trust Fund.

(Existing)

Reference: PSR 32 (1)

(d) Every inmate has at his disposal, while he is incarcerated, a prescribed percentage of his earnings, for use for authorized purchases. He shall have the remainder, after his contributions to the Inmate Welfare Fund, to the cost of goods and services provided to him and to income tax, where applicable, have been deducted, placed in a trust fund for him as compulsory savings.

(Conferred)

Reference: CD 232

(e) Every inmate has the right to request permission to use part of his savings money, while he is incarcerated, for purposes closely associated with his rehabilitation.

(Conferred)

Reference: CD 232

(f) No moneys in the Inmate Trust Fund that stand to the credit of an inmate shall be paid out unless:

(i) the inmate gives a direction in writing authorizing the payment out, and

(ii) the institutional head or other authorized officer certifies that, in his opinion, the payment is calculated to assist in the reformation and rehabilitation of the inmate.

(Existing)

Reference: PSR 32 (2)

(g) No moneys in the Inmate Trust Fund standing to the credit of an inmate shall, except where a family relationship exists, be transferred to the credit of another inmate.

(Existing)

Reference: PSR 32 (3)

(h) Every inmate shall receive interest on the funds in his inmate trust account.

(Conferred)

Reference: CD 210

# INJURIES AND DISABILITY

14. (a) Where an inmate sustains an injury, the matter shall be reported immediately to the medical staff for appropriate action.

(Conferred)

Reference: CD 207

(b) When an inmate suffers bodily injury, the institutional head shall cause an inquiry to be made and shall report to the Commissioner:

(i) the evidence taken on the inquiry;

(ii) the findings of the inquiry, and

(iii) the recommendation, if any, arising out of the inquiry.

(Existing)

Reference: PSR 33

(c) Subject to and in accordance with any regulations made under subsection 29 (1) of the Penitentiary Act, the Minister may pay compensation:

(i) to a discharged inmate for physical disability attributable to his participation in the normal program of a penitentiary, and

(ii) to the surviving spouse or dependent children of:

(a) a discharged inmate, or

(b) an inmate who died before the expiration of his sentence whose death is attributable to his participation in the normal program of a penitentiary.

In this section "discharged inmate" means an inmate who has been released as a result of the expiration of his sentence or the operation of remission or who has been released on parole other than day parole.

(Existing)

Reference: Penitentiary Act 28.1 (1)

# COMMUNICATION

15. Every inmate may, in accordance with the rules set out in Commissioner's Directives:

(a) communicate with persons or groups outside the penitentiary, and receive communication, except where there are grounds to believe that this would endanger the safety, security or well- being of others. This right carries with it special responsibilities and may therefore be subject to restrictions which are necessary (a) for the respect of the rights or reputations of others, or (b) for the security of the institution and the protection of individuals, or of public health or morals.

(Conferred)

Reference: CD 226

(b) engage in legitimate forms of personal expression, both alone and with others, except where there are grounds to believe that this would endanger the safety, security and well-being of others.

(Conferred)

Reference: CD 226

# NOTIFICATION OF ILLNESS OR DEATH

16. (a) Every inmate may inform his next of kin or closest known relative of his admission to a penitentiary, his transfer to another penitentiary, his serious illness, or of his transfer for treatment of mental illness. Should the inmate be incapable of making the communication himself, the information shall be communicated to the next of kin or closest known relative by the institutional authorities, providing that the inmate has signified, in writing, on or shortly after admission that he wishes them to be notified.

(Conferred)

Reference: CD 226

(b) Where an inmate dies while in custody, the institutional head shall forthwith inform the next of kin or closest known relative of the deceased.

(Existing)

Reference: PSR 34.(1)(a)

(c) Every inmate shall be informed as promptly as conditions permit of the death or serious illness of a family member as defined in CD 226 and may apply for temporary absence related to this situation in accordance with Directives.

(Conferred)

Reference: CD 226

# VISITS AND CORRESPONDENCE

17. Insofar as practicable the censorship of correspondence shall be avoided and the privacy of visits shall be maintained but nothing herein shall be deemed to limit the authority of the Commissioner to direct or the institutional head to order censorship of correspondence or supervision of visiting to the extent considered necessary or desirable for the reformation and rehabilitation of inmates or the security of the institution.

(Existing)

Reference: PSR 28

# INMATES' BUSINESS OPERATIONS

18. (a) (i) No inmate shall conduct a business while he is in custody unless he first obtains the approval of the Commissioner or other officer designated by the Commissioner.

(ii) The Commissioner or an officer designated by him under subsection (i) may grant approval under that subsection subject to such conditions as to the Commissioner or that officer seem appropriate and may at any time withdraw such approval.

(Existing)

Reference: PSR 25 (1) and (2)

(b) Notwithstanding subparagraph (a) above, an inmate shall be allowed an opportunity and reasonable assistance to wind up his business or have it operated on his behalf.

(Existing)

Reference: PSR 25 (3)

# APPEARANCE IN COURT

19. Where, pursuant to a judicial process, an inmate is required to give evidence in judicial proceedings in Canada, whether or not those proceedings are being conducted in the same territorial division as that in which the inmate is confined, the institutional head shall make available the inmate concerned for that purpose, if the party to the proceedings that requires the inmate:

(a) pays to the institutional head the cost of transportation, maintenance and custody for the inmate while he is absent from the institution pursuant to the process, or

(b) where the inmate is required by the Crown, undertakes to provide or to pay the cost of transportation, maintenance and custody for the inmate while he is so absent.

(Existing)

Reference: PSR 26

# DISCIPLINE

20. (a) Every inmate who is charged with a serious or flagrant disciplinary offence shall be treated fairly in accordance with the procedures laid out in the appropriate directives as they relate to the notification of charges, the conduct of hearings, the calling of witnesses, the recording of evidence and other matters.

(Conferred)

Reference: CD 213

(b) No inmate shall be punished except pursuant to:

(i) an order of the institutional head or an officer designated by the institutional head;

(ii) an order of disciplinary Court.

(Existing)

Reference: PSR 38.(2)

(c) Every inmate has a right to be free, under any circumstances, from cruel and unusual treatment or punishment.

(Retained)

Reference: Canadian Bill of Rights 2

(d) Where an inmate is convicted of a disciplinary offence the punishment shall, except where the offence is flagrant or serious, consist of loss of privileges.

(Existing)

Reference: PSR 38.(3)

(e) The punishment that may be ordered for a flagrant or serious disciplinary offence shall consist of one or more of the following:

(i) forfeiture of statutory remission or earned remission or both:

(ii) dissociation for a period not exceeding thirty days:

(iii) loss of privileges.

(Existing)

Reference: PSR 28.(4)

(f) Every inmate, who having been credited with statutory remission, is convicted in disciplinary court of any disciplinary offence is liable to forfeit, in whole or in part, the statutory remission that remains to his credit, but no such forfeiture of more than thirty days shall be valid without the concurrence of the Commissioner or an officer of the

Service designated by him, nor more than ninety days without the concurrence of the Minister.

(Existing)

Reference: Penitentiary Act 22.(3)

(g) Every inmate who, having been credited with earned remission, is convicted in disciplinary court of any disciplinary offence is liable to forfeit, in whole or in part, the earned remission that stands to his credit and that accrued after the coming into force of this section, but no such forfeiture of more than thirty days shall be valid without the concurrence of the Commissioner or an officer of the Service designated by him, or more than ninety days without the concurrence of the Minister.

(Existing)

Reference: Penitentiary Act 24.1(1)

# INTERVIEWS

21. Every inmate has the right, in accordance with the rules set out in Commissioner's Directives:

(a) (i) to be provided with a reasonable opportunity for an interview with the Commissioner of Corrections, when the Commissioner is visiting the institution, and when the inmate appears to have a legitimate ground of complaint, or when it appears that he might be assisted as a result of such an interview;

(Existing)

Reference: PSR 22.(1)

(ii) to be provided with a reasonable opportunity for an interview with the institutional head when he wishes to be heard.

(Existing)

Reference: PSR 22.(2)

(b) Every inmate shall be allowed:

(i) to have private interviews with the Correctional Investigator or his staff, at their request.

(Conferred)

Reference: CD 240

(ii) to have interviews, in private, with his legal counsel or any inspecting officer upon request, where safety and security conditions permit

(Conferred)

Reference: CD 226

# MEANS OF REDRESS

22. Every inmate has the right, in accordance with directives,

(a) to have access to a system set up for the redress of his grievances;
(Conferred)

Reference: CD 241

(b) to make complaints to the Correctional Investigator;
(Conferred)

Reference: CD 240

(c) to use privileged correspondence to communicate with designated officials.
(Conferred)

Reference: CD 219

# NON-PUNITIVE DISSOCIATION

23. (1) Where the institutional head is satisfied that:

(a) for the maintenance of good order and discipline in the institution, or

(b) in the best interests of an inmate, it is necessary or desirable that the inmate should be kept from associating with other inmates, he may order the inmate to be dissociated accordingly, but the case of every inmate so dissociated shall be considered, not less than once each month, by the appropriate institutional Board for the purpose of recommending to the institutional head whether or not the inmate should return to association with other inmates.

(2) An inmate who has been dissociated is not considered under punishment unless he has been sentenced as such and he shall not be deprived of any of his privileges and amenities by reason thereof, except those privileges and amenities that:

(a) can only be enjoyed in association with other inmates, or

(b) cannot reasonably be granted having regard to the limitations of the dissociation area and the necessity for the effective operation thereof.
(Existing)

Reference: PSR 40

# INTERNATIONAL AFFAIRS

24. (a) Every inmate who is a foreign national has the right, in accordance with the rules set out in Commissioner's Directives, to have the consular representatives of the State which takes charge of his interests, informed of his incarceration, to communicate himself with the consular representative, and to request to be visited by him. The

same right shall apply to an inmate who is a refugee or a stateless person, with respect to the representatives of the national or international authority whose task it is to protect him.

(Conferred)

Reference: CD 226

(b) A foreign offender may request transfer to a foreign state by applying to the Minister and may be transferred if the conditions set out in the Canadian Transfer of Offenders Act are met.

(Existing)

Reference: Transfer of Offenders Act 19.

# DISCHARGE

25. Where an inmate is discharged, he shall be given, in accordance with directives:

(a) at public expense, an issue of civilian clothing suitable to the season and other necessities,

(b) travelling and living expenses, at public expense, to:

(i ) the place where he was convicted.

(ii ) another place not further distant, if he so elects, or

(iii) any place in Canada, with the special approval of the Commissioner and,

(c) the moneys standing to his credit in the accounts of the institution.

(Existing)

Reference: PSR 21

# DEATH

26. (1) Where an inmate dies while in custody, the institutional head shall forthwith inform:

(a) the next of kin or closest known relative of the deceased,

(b) the coroner having jurisdiction in the area, and

(c) the Commissioner.

(2) Where the next of kin or closest known relative of the deceased does not claim the body of the deceased, it shall be decently interred, at public expense, in accordance with the rites of the religious faith of the deceased, but the cost of interment shall be charged against any money held in trust for the inmate.

(3) The body or any part of the body of a deceased inmate may be de-

livered to a recognized medical school or licensed hospital if the deceased, prior to his death, bequeathed his body or that part thereof for scientific purposes.

(4) The personal effects and money held in trust for a deceased inmate shall, subject to any lawful charges, be sent to his next of kin.

(Existing)

Reference: PSR 34